ELDER CARE

CHOOSING & FINANCING LONG-TERM CARE

BY JOSEPH MATTHEWS

EDITED BY BARBARA KATE REPA

please read this

We have done our best to give you useful and accurate information in this book. But please be aware that laws and procedures change constantly and are subject to differing interpretations. If you are confused by anything you read here, or if you need more information, check with an expert. Of necessity, neither the author nor the publisher of this book makes any guarantees regarding the outcome of the uses to which this material is put. The ultimate responsibility for making good decisions is yours.

access
NOLO
PRESS
to law

NOLO PRESS ■ 950 PARKER STREET
BERKELEY CA 94710 ■ 415/549-1976

printing history

Nolo Press is committed to keeping its books up-to-date. Each new printing, whether or not it is called a new edition, has been revised to reflect the latest law changes. This book was printed and updated on the last date indicated below. You might wish to call Nolo Press (415) 549-1976 to check whether there has been a more recent printing or edition.

New **PRINTING** means there have been some minor changes, but usually not enough so that people will need to trade in or discard an earlier printing of the same edition. Obviously, this is a judgment call and any change, no matter how minor, might affect you.
New **EDITION** means one or more major, or a number of minor, law changes since the previous edition.

FIRST EDITION	April 1990
EDITOR	Barbara Kate Repa
BOOK DESIGN	Jackie Clark
COVER DESIGN	Toni Ihara
INDEX	Sayre Van Young
PRINTING	Delta Lithograph

■ Nolo books are available at special discounts for bulk purchases for sales promotions, premiums, and fund-raising. For details contact: Special Sales Director, Nolo Press, 950 Parker Street, Berkeley CA 94710

Matthews, Joseph L.
    Eldercare : choosing & financing long-term care.

    1. Aged--Long term care--Evaluation. 2. Long-term care of the sick--Evaluation. 3. Aged--Long term care--Finance. 4. Long-term care of the sick--Finance. 5. Consumer education. I. Repa, Barbara Kate. II. Title.
RA644.5.M38 1990   362.1'6   90-7129
ISBN 0-87337-113-5

acknowledgments

Many thanks go to Ralph Warner, who saw immediately the value of a book such as this and who gave the project its birth.

Special thanks go to Peter Yedida, President of Geriatric Health Systems of San Francisco, who gave generously of his time and vast professional experience in matters of health care programs for the elderly. His corrective commentaries greatly strengthened the manuscript.

Special thanks also to Diane Arnold-Driver, Coordinator of the Center on Aging at the University of California, Berkeley. She shared readily her great expertise in geriatric care matters and tactfully made a number of suggestions which redounded to the significant benefit of the text.

A final and most exuberant thanks go to my editor, Barbara Kate Repa, whose perspicacity and skill are matched only by her patience and good humor. She needed all of them with me. The quality of this book is in large measure due to her talents.

RECYCLE YOUR OUT-OF-DATE BOOKS & GET 25% OFF YOUR NEXT PURCHASE!

Using an old edition can be dangerous if information in it is wrong. Unfortunately, laws and legal procedures change often. To help you keep up to date we extend this offer. If you cut out and deliver to us the title portion of the cover of any old Nolo book we'll give you a 25% discount off the retail price of any new Nolo book. For example, if you have a copy of TENANT'S RIGHTS, 4th edition and want to trade it for the latest CALIFORNIA MARRIAGE AND DIVORCE LAW, send us the TENANT'S RIGHTS cover and a check for the current price of MARRIAGE & DIVORCE, less a 25% discount. Information on current prices and editions is listed in the NOLO NEWS. Generally speaking, any book more than two years old is of questionable value. Books more than four or five years old are a menace. This offer is to individuals only.

OUT OF DATE = DANGEROUS

ELD 5/90

contents

chapter ten

BUYER BEWARE: NURSING HOME INSURANCE

appendix

RESOURCE DIRECTORY

MAKING DECISIONS ABOUT LONG-TERM CARE

MAKING DECISIONS ABOUT LONG-TERM CARE

A truth most everyone must face is that you or a family member will someday need some kind of expensive long-term care. Most older people, even if they remain basically healthy, develop physical or mental frailties or impairments which at some point prevent them from living completely independent lives. In 1989, over five million older people in the United States needed some form of daily at-home care provided by people outside the family.

Even more sobering is that half of all women and one-third of all men over age 65 will spend a part of their lives in some type of residential care facility. In 1989, for example, approximately 1.25 million people lived full-time in such facilities, at an average cost of $30,000 per year.

Medicare, often thought to "cover" medical care for everyone over 65, in fact pays for only about two per cent of all nursing facility costs. Medicaid, the federal government program which pays medical costs for the financially needy, pays for about half of all nursing facility costs, but it requires you to spend most of your personal assets before you can become eligible for coverage.

These statistics convey an urgent, unsettling message. This book's response to that message is to help you prepare for the likelihood of long-term care by presenting the alternatives you need to consider. The more physically, emotionally and financially comfortable you are, and the more in control of your own life, the better off you and your family will be.

A. WHAT IS LONG-TERM CARE?

As used in this book, "long-term care" means regular assistance with medical care (nursing, medicating, physical therapy) or personal needs (eating, bathing, moving around) provided by someone outside an older person's family. There are many varieties of long-term care—ranging from part-time home care, to adult daycare, to different levels of residential facilities. Some long-term care is temporary—for example, recovering from a broken hip or a stroke. More often, though, it lasts for the remainder of an older person's life: 25% of all nursing facility stays are for more than a year and many people are residents for two, three years or more.

B. COMPLEX QUESTIONS OF LONG-TERM CARE

An older person's debilitating condition may be only partial—such as failing hearing or eyesight, memory loss, partial paralysis. Or it may be extreme—the effects of a major stroke or Alzheimer's disease. Whatever the specific nature of the loss, the need for either temporary or permanent care raises a number of difficult questions:

- What kind of care is needed?
- Who will provide it?
- Where will it be provided?
- How much will it cost?
- Who will pay for it?

Attempting to answer these questions involves negotiating a number of consumer minefields: insurance rip-offs, unnecessary institutionalization, complicated Medicare and Medicaid rules, losing a home and assets to the high costs of nursing facilities or other care.

And if the elder is unable to arrange for the care needed, or is not fully aware of the need for care, the burden of providing care may fall heavily on other family members. Spouses and grown children often must take on major if not total responsibility for organizing and paying for long-term care. This book, then, is a guide not just for the elder who needs long-term care, but for all those who will participate in organizing, providing and paying for that care. The book emphasizes financial planning for long-term care: what Medicare and Medicaid pays for, how to protect an elder's assets from nursing facility costs, whether or not to purchase nursing facility insurance. The book also emphasizes the need to explore the many care alternatives to nursing homes and guides you in selecting a nursing home if that becomes necessary.

And the book explains legal devices and documents that can help protect an elder's dignity and ensure that wishes for medical procedures and property management are followed if he or she can no longer make decisions alone.

1. HOW THIS BOOK GUIDES YOU AND YOUR FAMILY

Many people, at many different stages in the process of deciding about how and where to get long-term care, will find guidance in this book.

- If your parent, grandparent or other older relative is no longer able to live a fully independent life, and you face questions of where additional care will come from, where your elder relative will live to receive that care, who will pay for it and how:

Of particular help to you may be the explanation in Chapter 2 of how a geriatric care manager can organize a program of care for your relative, especially if the elder lives in a different city or state from you. In addition, Chapters 3 and 4 discuss in detail how to choose the right kind and level of elder housing or nursing facility for your relative, and how to make sure the facility will provide a comfortable and humane residential setting.

Chapters 5 through 7 explain how much you can expect Medicare, Medicaid and other government programs to pay for long-term care, and how much of your relative's assets and income he or she will be able to retain or transfer to others. Throughout the book you will also find referrals to agencies and organizations that can provide detailed information and assistance about specific long-term care needs; this information is also collected in a Resource Directory in the Appendix of the book.

- If you or a family member are over fifty and want to begin planning to protect your home and other assets from the potential financial disaster of future long-term care:

In addition to the chapters on Medicare and Medicaid financing, you will find several other chapters particularly valuable. Chapter 7 discusses how to prevent the high cost of long-term care from eating up your lifetime savings. Chapter 8 explores ways to preserve your dignity and to retain the most control over your life and property when you are no longer physically or mentally able to handle all your own affairs. Chapter 9 gives an overview of estate planning techniques that can be used to protect an elder's money and property. And Chapter 10 shows in detail the many pitfalls of private insurance policies that claim to "cover" nursing home costs.

- ■ If your spouse or partner has personal assistance or medical needs the two of you are no longer able to handle without outside help, whether or not your spouse or partner has recognized the need:

In addition to Chapters 2 and 3, you will find valuable information in Chapter 6, which describes how the Medicaid government assistance program works and how much in assets and income it allows each spouse to retain, and in Chapter 7, which describes how you can protect some of your assets within the Medicaid rules.

- ■ If you increasingly find that you cannot manage all your own personal or medical needs without outside assistance and you face an immediate need to organize long-term personal assistance or medical care:

Extremely helpful and encouraging are Chapter 2 which introduces the many kinds of care available to you at home as alternatives to entering a nursing facility, and Chapter 3 which discusses the kinds of housing available for seniors that might provide the right level of assistance for you without the tremendous expense and unnecessary restrictions of a nursing facility.

C. THE IMPORTANCE OF EXPLORING LONG-TERM CARE OPTIONS

Although the sudden onset of an illness or disability does not always permit much advanced planning for long-term care, this book encourages you to be the best comparison shopper possible. If you are able to explore alternatives before full-time residence in a nursing facility is required, you not only improve your chances of obtaining the best care available, you may also be able to save a great deal of money.

Being prepared and researching alternatives when choosing long-term care allows you to realistically assess what is needed, and to choose only the kind of care that is actually required. In this way, you can avoid the loss of independence and great cost that come with taking on more care than is needed. This is particularly true when some combination of home health care and personal assistance is sufficient to permit a person to remain at home instead of entering a residential nursing facility. When time permits, certain financial planning you can do *before* residence in a nursing facility becomes necessary may permit you to protect a lifetime of savings and other assets. And even when long-term care is imminent, a little planning can go a long way toward lowering costs and protecting assets.

Finally, but not least important, the more thorough you are, the greater the opportunity for everyone concerned to participate—particularly if the person who needs care is not easily able to investigate and make decisions on his or her own. With more alternatives, everyone involved will have greater emotional room to come to terms with the decisions to be made.

D. RECOGNIZING AND DISCUSSING THE SITUATION

If you are the one who needs care, you may find it hard to discuss it with others because it seems a blow to your self-esteem, a subject that means you are really "old." You may also be reluctant to begin a process of giving up some of your independence, and fearful of what it may mean to give up full control over your life. And when you know you need the help of your family, you may be reluctant to bring up the subject because you know it will mean adding burdens to their lives.

If you believe that someone else—a family member or other loved one—is in need of care, you may be reluctant to bring up the subject because it may seem like a challenge or an insult. And within the family there may be anxiety, guilt and wide differences of opinion about what care is needed and from where and from whom it should come. The first step in providing needed care is to overcome the reluctance to talk about it. Once the discussion has begun, the information in this book can be of great help in organizing and choosing the right kinds of care.

1. GETTING HELP FROM OTHERS

To get discussion underway and onto the right track, it is often best to look outside the family. An unrelated person can sometimes soothe ruffled family feathers, present a neutral opinion and offer solutions not considered by the family. Also, it's sometimes easier to reveal fears and other feelings to an outsider than to an involved family member.

The following are some of the people you can turn to for help in beginning to evaluate long-term care needs:

- Your personal physician is often a good person to start with, not necessarily to moderate discussions but to give a prognosis of medical needs and to refer you to others who may be helpful in making plans.

- Traditional word-of-mouth is still one of the best ways to begin tackling any new problem. Friends and neighbors whose opinions you trust, and who may have already faced similar situations, are often a good source of information. So, too, the people at your local senior center may know of sources for long-term care assistance. These word-of-mouth sources often let you know of "unofficial" personal care aides who would not be available through more formal channels.

- A clergy member may be able both to help directly and to refer you and your family to professionals who can introduce alternatives and coordinate planning.

- County family service agencies, Area Agencies on Aging or other senior information and referral services are experienced sources that can provide direct access to specific care providers as well as help you develop an overall care plan. These agencies can direct you to a counselor or social worker who specializes in long-term care for elders and who can help you begin your discussions and planning. (See the Resource Directory in the Appendix of this book.)

- Once discussions are underway and residence in a nursing facility is not absolutely necessary, many people make use of the services of a professional geriatric care manager to see what at-home and other supportive services are available and to organize care from different providers. (Geriatric care managers are discussed in detail in Chapter 2.)

■
_____

IMPORTANT

If you are a family member helping to plan for someone else's
care, bear in mind that the most essential participant in planning
long-term care is the person whose care is being considered.

2. ASSESSING MEDICAL NEEDS

Because a specific physical impairment is often what leads to the need
for long-term care, one of the first things to do is to get professional
advice about the kind of medical care needed. A personal physician is
often the first person to talk with, although he or she may refer you to
a geriatric specialist for further consultation. And, as with all serious
medical decisions, if you are not completely comfortable with the
physician's assessment, seek a second opinion.

Whether or not you have a personal or family physician, an
excellent resource to help assess medical needs is a geriatric screening
program. Local hospitals have them, as do community and county
health centers. As with most initial referral questions, if you have
trouble finding a geriatric screening program, check with the county
social service agency, local or Area Agency on Aging, or call the senior
referral number in the white pages of the phone book.

Some of the things that must be addressed when assessing an
older person's need for medical care are:

SPECIFIC MEDICAL REQUIREMENTS

The doctor or other health screening personnel can discuss the elder's
specific medical needs, such as monitoring and administering drugs, or
providing physical therapy, explain what is involved in providing them
and let you know who can do it. The doctor or health care worker can
also discuss the level of ongoing care that would be required to deliver
those medical services: family members supplemented by occasional
visits from home care aides, a more sophisticated home care program,
or various levels of residential nursing facility care.

CHANGES IN CARE OVER TIME

The doctor or other health care worker can also discuss the medical prognosis—that is, what the future is likely to hold: whether to anticipate a short or long recovery period, whether a condition is likely to remain fundamentally the same over a long period, or whether it will become worse over a short or long period. Knowing the likely developments in the medical condition will allow you to plan the right level of care and to allow for changes.

MENTAL DISABILITIES

A thorough geriatric screening and evaluation are particularly important when the need for care arises from what seems to be a mental impairment. An older person's physical problems may become much more difficult to manage because of added symptoms of forgetfulness, disorientation, or general listlessness.

Such changes are usually assumed to be the beginnings of a permanent loss of mental faculties: the onset of senility or the early stages of Alzheimer's disease, both of which require careful long-term care planning.

Sometimes, though, what is thought to be an irreversible loss of mental facilities is really the result of some specific and treatable problem such as improper or over-medication, poor nutrition, depression about the loss of a spouse or a friend or about a physical disability, or a subtle medical condition that has not been diagnosed and treated. It is very important that a temporary and treatable loss of mental capacities is not misunderstood and perpetuated as a permanent condition.

In determining the true nature and cause of any loss of mental faculties, family members and friends can be particularly helpful to physicians and other health workers. The people who see an older person frequently are in the best position to know what factors may be contributing to diminished mental capabilities.

3. ASSESSING PERSONAL NEEDS AND CAPABILITIES

Equally as important but usually more difficult than assessing medical needs is determining what sort of personal, non-medical care is needed and what aspects of daily life a person can still manage without outside assistance. The question of the need and ability to care for oneself is not simply a matter of physical competence. Often, it is just as much about personality and emotional state. So, in addition to what kind of care is needed and the providers who are available and affordable, the ultimate decisions should depend a great deal on how important it is to the elder to remain in control of his or her own life.

Some people fiercely hold on to personal independence and privacy. For these people, who also have the ability to organize, manage and pay for individual programs to meet their specific needs, staying at home and receiving only minimal outside assistance may be both possible and extremely important.

Others may be willing to have an outside agency organize a more comprehensive care program, as long as they or their family members remain in primary control of daily life. For these people, an agency-directed program of home care in a family residence or in secured housing, perhaps combined with adult daycare, may be most appropriate if there are also family members willing to give additional assistance.

Still other people, however, prefer the security and ease of complete care organized and provided by others. For them, a residential care facility may be best, even though they may not physically require the high level of care offered there.

E. MAKING A REALISTIC FAMILY COMMITMENT

The options older people have to receive long-term care while maintaining their independence often depend on the extent to which family members are able and willing to help. But family situations vary widely in terms of relatives who can provide care, transportation, companionship or financial support to an elder. Before any long-term care program is organized—particularly when the elder is to remain at home without a spouse—family members must get together and discuss what sort of commitment each is willing to make to meet those needs that cannot be met by outside care.

Some of the possible arrangements requiring different levels of family involvement are:

1. STAYING AT HOME

The degree to which older people who need long-term care can maintain themselves in their own homes or apartments may depend on several kinds of family help. There may be a need for daily or weekly assistance with personal or medical care that is not provided by a home care or other outside agency. Help with housekeeping, shopping and home maintenance may be needed. And there will certainly be a need for regular visits and other help such as transportation to allow the elder to maintain contact with the outside world. Help may also be needed in planning, coordinating and overseeing outside care programs, as well as in planning and administering financial matters, including direct financial assistance.

2. MOVING IN WITH FAMILY

If older people needing long-term care are unable to maintain themselves in their own homes, they may still be able to avoid the cost and loss of independence of a residential care facility by moving in with willing family members and receiving long-term home care there. This kind of arrangement may permit family members to supplement home care provided by outside agencies with direct care of their own, keeping down costs and keeping up personal control.

But such an arrangement is obviously not for every family. It requires sufficient physical space and financial resources. And it takes the willingness of both the elder and the relatives with whom the elder lives. Everyone involved has to give up some room and some privacy and must make adjustments in daily habits and expectations. Relatives with whom the elder does not live must also be willing to share the responsibilities: visiting, outings, financial assistance. Obviously, all this takes a lot of talking, planning and ongoing cooperation among all family members.

3. ENTERING A RESIDENTIAL FACILITY

Recent surveys of nursing facility residents, have shown that contact with the world outside—leaving the facility for visits and outings, receiving visits, phone calls and mail from family and friends—is their single greatest concern. So even when an elder moves into an organized residential setting which provides personal care and social activities, or into a nursing facility which is supposed to provide complete care, family participation remains of the utmost importance.

To prepare for any residential care setting, family members must be willing to discuss both individually and as a group how much each is *realistically* able and willing to help. But most important, family members individually and collectively must discuss the future directly with the loved one who needs care.

F. THE ABILITY TO PAY

The information already discussed hints that planning to protect assets is important when considering a long-term care program or residential care facility. Fortunately, there are ways to protect some of your assets from nursing home costs and still receive Medicaid coverage. (See Chapter 7.) But many of the steps you can take must be accomplished before or immediately after entering a residential nursing facility. This points up why it is so important to start financial planning as soon as you begin considering long-term care—even though residence in a nursing facility may still be a long way off.

While many communities have a large number of care programs and residential facilities, almost all of them are quite costly. Home care, an alternative which can sometimes be less expensive than residential care, often runs $5,000 to $10,000 a year out of an elder's pocket—and many home care recipients pay even more. Residential nursing facility costs can be astronomical. In 1990, a nursing facility stay cost an average of $30,000 per year, with some nursing facilities running as high as $50,000.

Unfortunately, government programs and private insurance pay far less of these costs than most people think. Medicare pays only about two per cent of all nursing facility costs and precious little for home health care. (For a complete discussion of Medicare, Medi-gap and veterans' benefits, see Chapter 5.) Medicaid, the low-income federal medical support program, does pay about half of all nursing facility costs and a significant amount of home care charges. But Medicaid will begin paying only after you have used up most of your savings paying for your own care. (See Chapters 6 and 7.)

In fact, the cost of nursing facilities is so great that most people exhaust their life savings within six months of becoming a resident. What happens, then, if you remain in a nursing facility for a year? Two years? Four? What happens to your spouse who remains at home and needs those savings to live on? This book gives you the guidance you need to plan for these possibilities.

1. HELP WITH PAYING

In many places throughout this book, you will see references to coverage, and lack of coverage, of long-term care costs by Medicare, Medicaid and private insurance. Chapter 5 is devoted entirely to Medicare and private "Medi-gap" insurance coverage of long-term care; Chapter 6 covers Medicaid eligibility and coverage; Chapter 7 discusses how to protect personal assets and still qualify for Medicaid coverage and Chapter 10 covers nursing home insurance.

The following is a brief introduction to each subject so that you will be familiar with them as you read through the first few chapters on long-term care alternatives.

A BRIEF LOOK AT MEDICARE, MEDICAID AND INSURANCE

MEDICARE. Virtually everyone 65 and over is eligible.

Coverage for: Home care: 2 to 3 weeks; skilled nursing only; partial payment only

Senior residences: no coverage

Personal care facilities: no coverage

Nursing facilities: skilled nursing only; partial payment for periods up to 100 days, only if preceded by a hospital stay; only in facilities certified by Medicare

MEDI-GAP INSURANCE. Insurance policies must be purchased by each individual 65 or over.

Coverage for: Home care: usually no coverage; if any, only amounts Medicare does not pay for covered days

Senior residences: no coverage

Personal care facilities: no coverage

Nursing facilities: some policies cover, with same restrictions as Medicare, paying a part of what Medicare does not pay

MEDICAID [1]. Varies in each state; to be eligible you must have very low income and assets (not counting home, car and household goods).

Coverage for: Home care: personal as well as medical care; usually unlimited duration

Senior residences: not usually any coverage

Personal care facilities: extensive coverage in facilities certified by Medicaid; no time limit

Nursing facilities: extensive coverage at all care levels in certified facilities; no time limit

NURSING HOME INSURANCE. Private insurance policies purchased by individuals; they are expensive.

Coverage for: Home care: not usually covered; when it is, policies follow the same restrictions as Medicare, paying only what Medicare does not

Senior residences: no coverage

Personal care facilities: usually no coverage; when covered, many restrictions and small benefits

Nursing facilities: usually limited to skilled care; many restrictions; benefits depend on cost of policy and never cover full cost of nursing facility

---

[1]Called "Medi-Cal" in California.

2. DETERMINING INCOME AND ASSETS

The first step in assessing what money is realistically available for long-term care is to determine all income and available assets. For guidance, use the worksheet that follows which lists the most common categories of income, assets and liabilities. Fill in all the assets and income you know about. Consider the last category—Liabilities—as a set-off to be subtracted from available financial resources. Since this worksheet is informal, for your own reference, precise figures are not important. The worksheet is just intended to let you get a picture of the overall financial situation.

If you have a complete picture of income and assets, with the help of the information in Chapter 7 you can take steps to protect as many of those assets as possible against potentially catastrophic long-term costs.

When regular outside care does become necessary, determine which services and facilities might be at least partially covered by government programs or private insurance, and which are available at low or no cost.

Finally, involved family members must begin to think about their own financial contributions. While there may be no immediate need for money from relatives, the decisions made about long-term care may determine when money from beyond the elder's own resources will be required. The earlier this possibility is discussed, the easier it will be to plan and provide for it.

INCOME AND ASSETS WORKSHEET[2]

I. ESTIMATED INCOME
Ongoing business income   _____

Social Security retirement or disability benefits   _____

Pension benefits   _____

Income from rental property   _____

Income from patents or royalties   _____

Other income   _____

II. LIQUID ASSETS
Cash   _____

Savings and money market accounts   _____

Checking accounts   _____

Certificates of deposit   _____

U.S. savings and other bonds   _____

Gold, silver, rare coins and other precious metals   _____

III. PERSONAL PROPERTY ASSETS
Interest in ongoing business (ownership, stock option, profit-sharing)   _____

Value of any patents or copyrights   _____

Brokerage accounts and other stocks   _____

Money owed to you   _____

Automobiles, boats, other vehicles   _____

Antiques and works of art   _____

Valuable jewelry   _____

Face value of life insurance   _____

Miscellaneous   _____

IV. REAL ESTATE (FULL OR PARTIAL INTEREST)
Property #1 (current market value)   _____

Property #2   _____

Property #3   _____

V. LIABILITIES (WHAT YOU OWE)
Mortgage debts (all money you owe on real property listed above)   _____

Personal property debts (loans)   _____

Miscellaneous debts   _____

---

[2]As you fill out this worksheet, you may realize that your financial and ownership documents may be located in a number of different places. If so, this is a good time to gather them together and put them in one, safe place, then give a list of the documents and their location to family members or others you trust. *For the Record* (Nolo Press) is a computer program and manual that offer assistance in gathering and organizing this information.

AT-HOME CARE

chapter two

AT-HOME CARE

Until the 1970s, older Americans and their families had few choices when faced with elders' inability to care for themselves. The options were either family care at home or residence in a nursing facility or "rest home." Relying entirely on the family often placed an overwhelming burden on adult children and grandchildren and seriously strained family relations. Opting for care in a nursing facility, on the other hand, often created guilty feelings, seriously strained family finances, and at the same time restricted the elder's comfort and independence.

Fortunately, in recent years, a great increase in the number and kinds of home care services has meant that more elders who need care can either remain at home or live with relatives without putting undue stress on the family. The change has resulted in part from new technologies that make many medical treatments—such as oxygen and intravenous therapy—mobile enough for home administration.

Another impetus toward the home care option is the rapidly rising cost of residential nursing facility care, making consumers of medical care more interested in finding cost-effective alternatives. And in response to the larger number of people receiving medical care at home, agencies and programs have increased the kinds of therapeutic, nutrition, homemaking and other personal care services provided there.

This trend toward home care is particularly welcome given the fact that public health surveys indicate up to half of all nursing facility residents could live independently if they had adequate and affordable home care services. And other studies have shown that the longer people remain independent from institutional care, the better it is for their overall physical and emotional health.

Unfortunately, though, home care is currently practical only for people with a limited need for assistance—one that does not involve extensive medical treatment or continuous care. Home care may be sufficient if all one needs, for example, is help in getting exercise or physical therapy, monitoring a chronic health condition, or receiving meals. But if one needs several different kinds of care, or close monitoring for many hours of the day, the logistics and cost of home care may become prohibitive. In most cases, home care also requires family members who can fill in gaps it does not cover. For many people without such family assistance, home care is simply not an option.

■ ───────────────────────

HOME CARE NOW MAY STILL MEAN RESIDENTIAL CARE LATER

Even if home care is a workable alternative, you may well want to begin planning for the possibility of residence in a nursing facility at some later date. As discussed in detail in Chapter 7 proper financial planning can save you and your family thousands of dollars in the event a residential nursing facility becomes necessary. And several of the most effective tools for protecting your assets are available only if they are used well in advance of nursing home residence. Although limited home care may be all you need right now, the smartest planning for long-term care looks as far ahead as possible.

A. WHAT IS HOME CARE?

Home care encompasses a multitude of medical and personal services provided at home to a partially or fully dependent elder.[1] These services often make it possible for an older person to remain at home, or with a relative, rather than enter a residential facility for extended recovery or long-term care.[2] Depending on what is available in your community, home care and related supplemental services can include:

───────────────────────

[1]Although home care is available for people of any age who require long-term care, this book focuses on the needs of older people.

[2]In this book, the terms "home" and "home care" refer to the private house or apartment where the elder lives alone, with spouse or other family or friend. What used to be called "rest homes" and "nursing homes" are now generally referred to as "board and care facilities" and "nursing facilities."

- Health care—nursing, physical and other rehabilitative therapy, medicating, monitoring and medical equipment;
- Personal care—assistance with personal hygiene, dressing, bathing and exercise;
- Nutrition—meal planning, cooking, meal delivery or meals at outside meal sites;
- Homemaking—housekeeping, shopping, home repair service, household paperwork;
- Social and safety needs—escort and transportation services, companions, telephone check, overall planning and program coordination service.

(See Sections C and D below, for a complete discussion of the many available home care and related services.)

Not everyone using home care will need all of the services available, not every community will have every possible service and no single program or agency can provide everything that might be required. Additional needs may have to be filled by community agencies or organizations, adult daycare or senior centers, individuals hired through informal networks, family and friends.

1. INDEPENDENCE

One advantage of home care is that you and your family can better control the care you receive and avoid care you don't want or need. For home care to work well, though, you and your family must take the initiative to find services and coordinate different programs and personnel, monitor home care performance, figure costs and budgets and make changes when required. All of that can be a significant burden on top of meeting day-to-day needs for physical care.

2. FINANCIAL SAVINGS

In addition to the physical and emotional advantages of remaining at home, there can also be significant financial savings if the care required is not too complicated or frequent and family and friends supplement paid care. While residential care facilities average $15,000 to $50,000 a year, home care can average from 50% to 75% less, depending on what care is required. You save by not paying for unnecessary services or institutional overhead. The things you provide yourself at home—food, drugs, supplies—come without any nursing facility mark-up.

On the other hand, once care becomes extensive or complicated, the economies of scale may make residence in a nursing facility less expensive.

3. IS HOME CARE RELIABLE?

While these features of home care sound attractive, you may have lingering doubts about whether you can receive the same quality of care at home as you would in a nursing facility.

The American Medical Association, the American Hospital Association, the American Nurses' Association and the United States Government Department of Health and Human Services all endorse the quality of medical and nursing care delivered by home health care agencies that have been certified by both Medicare and by the state's home care licensing agency. Of course, you should consult your doctor before deciding whether to receive specific medical care at home, and your doctor should periodically review the quality of that care.

Remember, it is always important to be a responsible consumer, choosing a provider only after comparison shopping for the best quality and most cost-efficient care. If you do handle the decision carefully, you may be able to receive home care as good as, and often cheaper than, nursing facility care. And, by using different providers and changing when you aren't satisfied, you may be better able to control the quality of care you receive than in nursing facilities which allow for little or no choice.

B. HOW TO FIND HOME CARE SERVICES

As you've probably gathered by now, arranging a program of home care involves some searching and organizing, and often means using services from more than one source. To do this, you need to learn where to find these services and how to locate recommended agencies and individuals.

Much of home care—particularly nursing and other medical services—can be provided by a home care or home health care agency. (The services such agencies provide is discussed below in Section C.)

There are a number of ways to find one:

1. FRIENDS AND RELATIVES

While the opinions of professionals are often helpful, friends and relatives who have had home care experiences can be an excellent place to start. Informal information-sharing can reveal a program or person unknown to an agency or professional, and can warn you about providers to avoid despite their apparently sound credentials. Call a few friends or relatives and tell them the kind of help you think you need. They may be able to tell you of other people they know who have arranged for similar help. This kind of networking can snowball, with each phone call leading you to others to contact for information or services. Don't be shy. Call around and start the snowball rolling.

2. HOSPITAL PERSONNEL

If you are looking for home care following a stay in a medical facility, most have a "discharge planner" or "social services" administrator who can refer you to a home care agency capable of meeting your needs. Many hospitals and skilled nursing facilities operate their own home health care units. Although you should not automatically sign up with the hospital or nursing facility's home care unit, it is a good place to start comparison shopping.

3. PHYSICIANS

Your own physician may know of a good home care agency with which he or she has worked. That would offer the assurance that your doctor is willing to work with the particular agency. Your doctor may also be willing to put you in contact with other patients who use the agency.

4. NURSING REGISTRIES

If your need is primarily for at-home nursing, contact your local hospital, which probably has a registry of visiting nurses. The local chapter of the Visiting Nurses' Association provides visiting nurses and may also be a good source of referrals for other care.

5. NATIONAL, STATE AND LOCAL AGENCIES AND ORGANIZATIONS

If your need for home care is the result of a particular illness or disability, ask for referrals from the local chapter of a volunteer organization that focuses on that illness or disability, such as the American Heart Association, American Cancer Society, American Diabetes Association, the Alzheimer's Foundation, among others.

Many public agencies that specialize in the needs of older people can also refer you to home care agencies in your area. The federal government has set up A10

rea Agencies on Aging which operate some federally-funded programs which can be of direct help; the area agencies can also refer you to Medicare-approved home care agencies.

Most states, too, have their own Agencies on Aging—and there may be local offices of the state agency in your own community. Check the state government listings in the white pages of the telephone book.

City and county Agencies on Aging may have low-cost programs of their own and can also refer you to reputable home care agencies. Referral services can be found in your phone book under listings for Senior Referral, Department of Social Services, Family Service Agency, or Information and Referral. Often these services have a social worker or public health worker who specializes in referrals for older people.

■
_____

FOR MORE INFORMATION

For addresses and telephone numbers of many of these organizations and agencies, see the Resource Directory in the Appendix of this book.

6. SENIOR CENTERS

Because it is part of the job of local senior centers to provide information for seniors, they are usually happy to help with referrals to agencies and individual services. Home care providers know that senior centers supply this information, so they often make their services known at the centers. You can also get personal recommendations and opinions from other older people at the centers.

7. VOLUNTEER ORGANIZATIONS

A number of community volunteer organizations not only provide referrals, but also administer their own home care programs. Your local United Way, for example, is a good clearing house for different services. Churches or synagogues, and local religious, ethnic or fraternal agencies and organizations are often very helpful in coordinating home care services, usually free of charge, and in helping you make informal care arrangements.

■

OLDER PEOPLE HELPING OLDER PEOPLE

The Retired Senior Volunteer Program (RSVP) is a federally-funded program through which retired older people volunteer to help other less mobile elders. RSVP, together with the Senior Companion Program, provides all sorts of general assistance with non-medical daily needs, free of charge. And if RSVP is not equipped to help you directly, it may well be able to refer you to a program or agency that can. To find your local RSVP, look in the white pages of the phone book or contact the national office of ACTION, 1100 Vermont Avenue, NW, Washington, DC 20525, (800) 424-8867. The national office will help connect you with the branch nearest you.

8. GERIATRIC CARE MANAGERS

In the last several years, a new and potentially helpful field has developed, known as private care management for the aging, or geriatric care management. Care managers are professional counselors or guides who, either on a one-time or ongoing basis, help assess long-term care needs and organize services to meet those needs.

Geriatric care managers can assist with nursing facility placement, but they are most helpful in guiding you through the maze of home health care and other support services needed for long-term care in the home. They can be particularly useful when family members live in a different city from the person who needs the care. Care managers may know of difficult-to-find services; they can evaluate agencies and individual care givers; they can help set up a coordinated program of care among several providers; and they can follow-up with ongoing management and changes in care.

However, nothing as important as decisions about long-term care should be left solely in the hands of any one adviser. After all, the choices are not going to affect the care manager's life; they're going to affect yours. The more you know and the more you participate in decision-making, the better able you will be to choose among the alternatives a care manager can offer.

WHERE TO FIND GERIATRIC CARE MANAGERS

As with other long-term care resources, your personal physician, a local senior citizens center, or friends and neighbors might be able to refer you to geriatric care managers.

You can also find geriatric care managers in the white pages of the telephone directory under "Geriatric Care," "Geriatric Management," "Older Adults Care Managers," or something similar. Your local senior information or senior referral directory—usually listed separately in the white pages (sometimes under county or city offices or public health department) can also make referrals. Several national organizations, including Aging Network Services, can help locate care managers in your area. (Addresses and telephone numbers for these organizations can be found in the Resource Directory in the Appendix of this book.)

EVALUATING A GERIATRIC CARE MANAGER

There is no easy way to know in advance whether a particular geriatric care manager is reputable and effective. Good care managers sometimes work on their own, sometimes with an organization dedicated to care management. Unfortunately, there are no firm guidelines and no state certifications yet for this relatively new field. Here are some ideas, though, on what to ask before hiring a geriatric care manager:

- Where has the care manager worked before? Experience with a local public agency that deals with the elderly is a good sign, as is work with a local nursing facility or home health care agency. Whatever the form, some public health experience is essential. The care manager should provide you with references from previous employment if you ask for them.

- What is the care manager's professional training? Normally, a care manager should have a license or degree in public health nursing, public health management, social work or gerontology. If not, be very sure that the person has an extensive work history you can check personally.

- Does the care manager belong to any state or national professional organizations? Membership in a professional organization such as the National Association of Social Workers, Visiting Nurse Association or National Association of Private Geriatric Care Managers does not guarantee quality of work, but it may indicate a professional attitude and a willingness to have credentials verified.

- How does the care manager structure fees? Find out in advance exactly what you will be charged for and how much. Some organizations operating with public or philanthropic support offer free or low-cost services to low-income individuals and families. With many private care managers there is a flat fee ($100 to $250) for the initial family visit and evaluation, then an hourly charge ($15 to $100) for making arrangements and for follow-up visits. Whatever the terms, make sure to get them in writing.

- How extensive is the follow-up? After initial arrangements have been made, to what extent is the care manager available for personal or telephone consultations? For emergencies? What are the charges? Are there continuing services available, such as weekly or monthly reviews or visits, either by phone or in person? And what happens if a service or provider the care manager has arranged for does not work out? On what terms will the care manager arrange for replacement services?

■ Does the care manager have any clients or former clients who can give a personal recommendation? Speaking with someone who has used the care manager's services before may give you both confidence in the care manager and a better idea of what to expect.

■ _____

REMEMBER

Relying on a care manager should not stop you from also checking with friends and relatives or otherwise looking for care on your own.

C. SERVICES PROVIDED THROUGH HOME CARE

Home care services range from covering the most obvious needs of the older person—help with medication, therapy and special equipment— to respite care that gives a break to the usual care providers.

1. MEDICAL SERVICES

Most home care agencies as well as Visiting Nurses' Associations can provide or arrange for a number of medical services, including skilled and basic nursing, rehabilitation therapies and dietary services.

NURSING

With a physician overseeing the course of treatment, a home care agency or nursing registry can provide geriatric nurse practitioners, registered nurses and licensed vocational or practical nurses. These highly skilled nurses plan and monitor health care, give injections and intravenous medication and instruct you on self-administered medications, injections and treatments.

More routine nursing care is provided by vocational and practical nurses and by aides who work under the nurses' supervision. They monitor pulse, blood pressure and temperature and administer simple diagnostic procedures, such as drawing blood and other samples for the laboratory and instruct home patients on how to use portable testing equipment.

THERAPIES

Most home care agencies provide a physical therapist, respiratory therapist, speech therapist or occupational therapist. These specialists give short-term assistance to people recovering from an illness or injury and ongoing therapy to those with permanent disabilities.

NUTRITION

Most agencies also either have someone on staff or can arrange for someone to help plan a diet and show how to prepare foods that provide proper nutrition and meet special dietary needs. Help in shopping for and preparing meals may also be available, as are meals brought in fully prepared.

2. MEDICAL AND SAFETY EQUIPMENT AND SUPPLIES

Home care agencies can provide medical equipment and supplies such as a hospital bed, wheelchair, walker, oxygen equipment and various home testing and monitoring equipment, as well as supplies for incontinence and other conditions. The equipment can be either bought or rented from the agency or from a medical equipment company with which the agency does business.

Some home care agencies can also inspect your home for safety needs and arrange to install any necessary equipment, such as support railings, access ramps or an emergency response system.

■

A NOTE ON SAVING MONEY

Find out whether you are required to buy or rent all medical equipment and supplies from any home care agency you are considering. If so, and you need substantial medical equipment or supplies, make sure their prices are competitive with what you would pay if you purchased the equipment or supplies on your own. Always comparison shop before buying equipment or having any work done through an agency.

3. NON-MEDICAL PERSONAL CARE

Many people do not need skilled medical care as much as assistance with personal tasks that have become difficult because of frailty or other physical debility. This is provided not by skilled medical personnel, but by "home health aides" or "home care aides."

Aides are the people who spend the most time with you. Their tasks vary, depending on your needs and on the rules of the agency or willingness of the individual aide, but in general they include:

- assistance with personal care such as bathing, grooming, toilet needs, eating;
- help with movement or exercise, such as getting around the house, stretching, taking a walk;
- simple health tasks, such as taking blood pressure and temperature and helping with self-administered medications, salves and breathing equipment; and
- minimal homemaking, such as helping to plan and cook simple meals.

More general homemaking services (grocery shopping, meal preparation and clean-up, light housecleaning and laundry) are often available through home care agencies, but they are provided by different personnel and may be charged differently from a home health aide's visit. Not every home care agency provides homemaking services, however, and you may need to make separate arrangements through informal networks of friends, relatives and neighbors.

■
_____

REMEMBER TO ASK

Just because something is not on a home care agency's or
individual aide's list of offered services does not mean it is not
available. Depending on how flexible your home care aide is,
any light task around the house might be included. If the aide
will not help, or is not allowed by an agency to assist with
certain needed tasks, the agency may be able to provide
someone who can.

RESPITE CARE

With home care, the primary responsibility for care and companionship
often still rests with family members. Particularly when an elder
requires extensive monitoring, that can become a substantial burden on
family members who must stay around the house. Some agencies
provide temporary respite care—a companion for the elder, whose
presence allows a family member to leave the house and go to work,
attend to other business, or simply have a break. Obviously, you can
also make private arrangements for someone to fill this need.

Respite companions are often volunteers, organized through a
community group. If your agency does not have respite care, it should
be able to refer you to a community group or organization that does
provide it. (See Section H, Supplements to Home Care, below.)

D. KINDS OF HOME CARE PROVIDERS

Home care providers range from hospitals or other high-tech
organizations with highly trained medical staffs, to full-service home
care agencies, to the ten year-old kid down the block who takes out
your trash. Getting the most sophisticated and well-equipped home
care provider is not the point. The goal is to find providers who can
bring you the specific care you need, and no more, for the best price.

1. FULL-SERVICE HOME CARE AGENCIES

Most home care agencies, whether their name refers to general home care or specifically to home *health* care, provide a great variety of services. Some agencies offer more services than others, although a few will supply all the services mentioned below. Some will help you find outside services they don't provide; others will leave it to you to fill in gaps. In any case, if there is a service you may need that the agency does not mention, be sure to ask about it. If an agency cannot provide the service, it may know someone who can.[3]

Home care agencies are often affiliated with hospitals, nursing facilities and nursing organizations. But since most home care is *not* direct medical care, the fact that an agency is connected with a medical institution does not necessarily mean it will provide better overall personal care.

On the whole, full-service agencies tend to be more expensive than independent providers or support-care agencies that do not provide nursing or medical therapies. Despite their higher cost, though, they can be extremely useful when it is necessary to coordinate different levels of care and there are no family members available to organize and oversee separate independent providers.

2. SUPPORT-CARE AGENCIES

Support-care agencies provide personal, household and respite care, but not skilled nursing or medical therapies. They are often sponsored by community or charitable organizations and because they do not maintain highly skilled medical staffs, some can provide home aides at lower rates than full-service agencies. (In choosing a support care agency, refer to the criteria discussed in Section E, What to Look for in a Home Care Agency.)

---

[3]Many home care agencies will create a written care plan and provide a written estimate of costs as part of any contract you sign for their services. Review the care plan and contract carefully to make sure you are not obligated to buy, rent or pay for any services or equipment in the future.

3. INDEPENDENT AND INFORMAL ARRANGEMENTS

As emphasized throughout this chapter, not all care must come through a formal agency. More important, not all *good* care comes from an agency. Independent home care workers are often more flexible in the tasks they will perform, and are also less expensive, than agency personnel.

FINDING INDEPENDENT AIDES

Some communities have what are called In-Home Support Services that refer home attendants and aides for non-medical home care. And many public agencies, community or charitable organizations and churches,[4] while not sponsoring a home care agency, offer a referral list of independent home care aides the organization or agency vouches for and has referred successfully in the past.

Professional nurses and nonprofessional aides can also be found through informal networks. Friends and relatives may know of an individual who suits your needs but who does not work through an agency and may not have any formal certification or training. Many people have found that "unofficial" aides provide very personal, flexible and competent assistance and charge considerably less than certified nurses or aides.

Keep in mind, though, that the range and quality of care you get depends entirely on the knowledge, skill and attitude of the one caregiver. There is no outside supervision, no one to compare the quality of care you are getting with the quality you should be getting. Also, with an independent aide, no agency has checked into the background of the person who will be spending a considerable amount of time in your home. And while agencies routinely post a "bond" for their aides to protect the consumer from theft or damage by the home care aide, most independent aides are not bonded.

Finally, a common and significant problem with independent aides arises when they are sick or otherwise unavailable. If you will

---

[4]Some churches in areas with large immigrant populations attempt to help both their churchgoers in need of home care and undocumented immigrant workers by referring the undocumented immigrants as home care aides. These undocumented aides are badly in need of work and therefore provide home care at a lower price than "official" aides. If you are in a real financial pinch, and the home care you require is not skilled medical care, you may want to contact your local church about such aides.

need an independent aide regularly, it is a good idea to have a back-up
to call on short notice.

■
_____

HOME CARE PERSONNEL

Different types of care are provided by home care agency
workers with different titles and skills. Knowing the types of
personnel can help you make use of the services an agency has
to offer. Also, because fees are higher for more skilled workers,
understanding the different categories can help you avoid having
an *overqualified*, and therefore overly expensive, home care
provider when a less skilled but equally effective provider is also
available.

Supervisors and Planning Coordinators:
Probably the first person you will have contact with, the planner
assesses your needs and capabilities and develops an overall
plan for care. The planner may also oversee personnel
assignments, and if so, may be the one to consult about changes
in services or personnel after your care has begun.

Clinical or Nursing Supervisors: A clinical
supervisor, usually a public health or geriatric nurse, monitors
your direct home medical care, including diet and nutrition. This
is the person for you, your family or your doctor to speak with if
you have a question or problem with the skilled medical care
you receive.

Social Workers: The agency's social worker, resource
manager or caseworker can help coordinate your care with other
programs and services not provided by the agency and can help
with financial and insurance planning and paperwork.

Nurses: Every home health care agency should have at
least one nurse practitioner or registered nurse (RN) on call at all
times to monitor patient nursing needs. Nurse practitioners
generally supervise other nurses, and can prescribe some
medicines, give injections and diagnose routine medical
problems. Registered nurses handle complex nursing functions,
including administering intravenous medication, drawing blood
and making an overall assessment of patient needs and a nursing
care plan to meet those needs.

A Licensed Vocational Nurse (LVN) or Licensed Practical Nurse (LPN) handles the more routine nursing tasks, such as monitoring blood pressure and pulse, checking fluids, administering oxygen and some medications and doing some basic physical rehabilitation.

If you require a special physical rehabilitation program—after a hip injury or a stroke, for example—a Certified Rehabilitative Nurse (CRN) may plan the program, begin you on it and monitor your progress, sometimes in conjunction with a rehabilitation therapist.

Rehabilitation Therapists. Physical, occupational, speech and respiratory therapists plan and carry out a program of rehabilitative therapy. Once you are on a regular program, routine therapy assistance is often handled by trained assistants or technicians.

Home Care Aides. The home care aide is the foot soldier of home care. The aide handles simple, everyday health and personal care tasks: bathing, grooming, moving around, exercising, helping with self-administered medications, creams and therapies, monitoring blood pressure and temperature. The aide may also help you with minimal homemaking—planning and preparing simple meals, some amount of home organizing. But the home care aide is *not* a housekeeper or house cleaner; these services may or may not be available through your home care agency. An independent home care aide, on the other hand, may be more flexible about a certain amount of household work.

Companions. Sometimes the greatest need one has, particularly if house-bound, is simply for company. Some home care agencies provide, often through a community group, people known as "companions," who will spend time in the home or go for a small outing—shopping, to the library, to the park or just for a walk—to give an elder some company and conversation. Companions may also help with personal paperwork, make phone calls and organize slightly more complicated outings.

E. WHAT TO LOOK FOR IN A HOME CARE AGENCY

Although you may find good quality and less expensive care without using a home care agency, if you do choose to use one, here are some of the things to look for:

1. CERTIFICATION

This is not a guarantee of quality care, but a full-service agency should be approved by both Medicare and your state's Medicaid program. The government checks to make sure certain staff, supervision and basic training requirements are met. Likewise, if your state licenses home care agencies, make sure your agency has such a license. To find out, call your area or local Agency on Aging. (See the Resource Directory in the Appendix.)

Also, some agencies are accredited by national health care organizations. For example, the Joint Commission for Accreditation of Health Care Organizations is the umbrella organization that accredits home health care agencies.

2. REPUTATION

Here are some questions to ask:

- How long has the agency been in business? Look for an agency that has stood the test of time.
- Does the agency belong to the National Association of Home Care or to a state home care association? Membership may indicate adherence to certain standards of care.
- Can the agency give references to doctors and public health workers who have worked with the agency and to clients? Talk directly with the references, and if medical care is involved, try to have your doctor do so, too.

3. SERVICES AND FLEXIBILITY

No matter how many services an agency claims to offer in its brochure, the important thing is to match its services with your needs. And if you have any special scheduling needs, make sure the agency will accommodate you. Also, find out if there is any extra cost for night or weekend services.

Flexibility in care is also very important. An agency may be able to meet your needs at first, but what if your needs change? Can the agency also provide different, more specialized medical services, a more unusual schedule, household work? It is not necessary that the agency *directly* provide every service you might need in the future, as long as it has the capacity to arrange the service through coordination with other providers.

Before choosing an agency, ask the planning coordinator about the availability of other services. What are their regular arrangements with other programs or agencies? What is the extra charge for such services? Can they arrange for services which they do not already have on call?

4. PERSONNEL STANDARDS

Find out about an agency's personnel before you begin to receive care. What are the skill levels of both in-home and planning personnel on staff? What training and experience are required for different positions? Even non-medical home care aides should have completed some formal training.

Since home care workers will be spending a significant amount of time in your home, often with no one else present, find out what process the agency uses to screen an employee's background.

5. WHAT DOES *NOT* MATTER IN CHOOSING
   AN AGENCY

Some things about home care agencies may seem to be important considerations in choosing a home care agency, but in fact are not important.

NONPROFIT, CHURCH-RELATED OR CHARITABLE ORGANIZATION

Because an agency is "nonprofit," will it be less expensive? Or if the agency is sponsored or owned by a church or a charitable organization, will it have the client, rather than money or the appearance of doing good works, foremost in mind?

The answer to both questions is: not necessarily. Some organizations that operate home care agencies acquire nonprofit tax status by associating with a larger nonprofit group. This means they pay less in taxes, but it does not mean that the rates they charge will be cheaper; only a comparison of rates with other agencies can tell you that.

Nor does a nonprofit status mean the quality of care is any better. Just because a church or charitable organization sponsors an agency does not mean it has anything to do with the agency's daily operations. These are usually handled by an independent administration, and it is *their* work that determines the quality of care.

NATIONAL CHAIN

An agency that is part of a large nationwide organization may appear to have a better administration than a small, independent agency. In certain respects that may be true—for example, standardized personnel duties, or computerized billing may make some aspects of home care easier to manage. But gains in paper efficiency may be lost in personalized care. The quality of care you receive from any agency, national chain or small independent, depends on the skill and attention of the people who will be in your home giving you hands-on care.

HOSPITAL-CONNECTED

An agency affiliated with a hospital may appear better able to provide medical care than other agencies. But keep in mind that most home care does not involve complicated medical treatment. An agency that focuses on high technology health care may be giving too little attention to what most home care recipients need most—thoughtful human attention.

F. GETTING STARTED WITH HOME CARE

Whether or not you use the services of an agency, settling on a home care plan is an important first step. Your diligence may also be required in supervising the care and updating the care plan as needed.

1. DEVELOPING A CARE PLAN

If you are using an agency, personnel there should consult with you and your family in developing a plan, rather than imposing a pre-arranged care package on you.[5] And agency or not, since your family will probably be providing additional care, family members should be directly involved in planning.

If you have special needs—rehabilitative therapy or restricted diet, for example—then specialists in those areas should also participate in planning. And consultations with your doctor should also be a part of the development of a care plan. It is important for a home care plan to take into account your overall comfort and need for human contact as well as specific medical care—for example, providing aides who can speak a language you are comfortable speaking, or aides who do not smoke, if that is your preference. In search of such a match, an agency planner should make at least one extensive visit to the home where you will be receiving care *before* finalizing a plan. And although you will certainly be keeping an eye on your own financial limits, an agency planner should also take into account your financial capabilities.

If you are making up your own care plan, it may help you keep track to formulate a blueprint of services based on the suggested checklist below. Be sure to include family members and friends who will help with care as well as paid or volunteer outside aides.

---

[5]Some agencies automatically deliver more care than is needed, partly because the more services they provide, the more money they make. Not only does this raise costs unnecessarily, but for many people, receiving too much care stops them from doing things for themselves, which can be an important part of continued psychological well-being.

■ _____

CHECKLIST FOR HOME CARE PLAN

1. Medical and Rehabilitation Care:
   Service:
   —Provider:
   —When provided:
   —Additional non-professional:
   —Follow-up care (who & when):

2. Non-medical Care (including personal assistance, meals, homemaking, escort, companion, transportation, phone check):
   Service:
   —Provider:
   —When provided:

2. PROVIDING AND SUPERVISING CARE

A home care plan is only as good as the people who carry it out. In addition to the training and experience of home care personnel, something harder to evaluate—how well you get along—is also important. It helps to meet and interview home care aides *before* they begin to provide care. Although it can save everyone trouble later on, some agencies discourage advance selection to prevent clients from overshopping for the "perfect" aide.

Continuity of care givers is also important. Once you have developed a relationship with care givers who understand your needs, you want to be able to count on them regularly. On occasion, there are legitimate reasons, such as illness or vacation, for a temporary substitute. But even in these instances, substitute care should be provided only by an aide regularly employed by the agency and not by an independent or "freelance" care giver unless that person's qualifications and background have been subjected to the same scrutiny as regular employees.

3. SUPERVISION AND COMPLAINTS

If you use the services of a home care agency, that agency should regularly review the care plan. The original plan may not have addressed your needs adequately, your needs may have changed over time, or the people actually giving you care may not be doing their jobs properly.

A staff member skilled in the specific care involved should regularly supervise and review your care. A certified therapist should be checking on your therapy aide and a registered nurse should be checking on health care aides. The frequency of the reviews depends on the level of care. Medicare, for example, requires that a supervisor visit the home *at least every two weeks* if the care is for a chronic or acute illness. If there is no skilled medical care involved, home visits by supervisors can be less often—every four to eight weeks, perhaps—but a supervisor should be in at least weekly contact with the care giver.

There should be an easy way for you to register complaints with a supervisor about the care you are receiving. There should be frequent telephone contact between you and a supervisor, and there should also be regular in-person supervisor reviews of your care—with your family members present, if you wish.

G. COSTS OF HOME CARE

As discussed in detail in Chapters 5 and 6, you cannot count on Medicare or private insurance to pay for much of home care, and Medicaid will pay for some home care only if you have used up most of your own assets. Since payments will come primarily from your own pocket, pay close attention to the way a home care provider calculates its charges. Many agencies will give you a written estimate of charges based on the plan they develop with you. Before signing up, read this section carefully and then measure the true total charges against your income and assets.

■

GOVERNMENT-CERTIFIED PROVIDERS

Medicare and Medicaid Approved: Even if the care you receive initially is not covered by Medicare or Medicaid, or you are not eligible for Medicaid, make sure the agency or other provider is certified for both. Your physical situation may change, making your care eligible for Medicare coverage. (See Chapter 5.) Or your financial situation may change, making you eligible for Medicaid. (See Chapter 6.) If the agency is certified, you would be sure of continuity in your home care.

State Licensed: Some states have minimum quality standards and issue home care licenses or certificates to those agencies or individual providers that qualify. If you have private insurance that covers home health care, it usually requires a state-approved provider. (Insurance coverage for home care is discussed in detail in Chapter 5.)

1. SLIDING SCALE (INCOME-BASED) FEE POLICY

Many public agency, community, church and philanthropic organization home care providers base eligibility and fees on the care recipient's income. In other words, you only qualify if your income is below a certain level and the lower your income, the lower the charge. These are not always full-service home care agencies, but if they can meet your needs, they may offer significant savings for you.

2. COST VARIES WITH SERVICE AND SKILL LEVEL

Most agencies and individual providers charge by the hour or by the visit. Agencies sometimes also have a minimum daily or weekly charge. Generally, the amount charged reflects the skill level of the provider. It therefore makes sense not to receive simple care from a highly skilled provider when someone less skilled can provide it just as well. Roughly, rates are divided as follows:

- nurse practitioners and registered nurses, $50 to $100 per hour
- practical and vocational nurses, licensed rehabilitative therapists and geriatric social workers, $35 to $75 per hour

- home health aides, $10 to $20 per hour
- homemakers, home workers and companions, $7 to $15 per hour

Note: The rates charged by independent care givers are usually lower than those charged by agencies. The rates also vary in different parts of the country.

3. BEWARE THE HIDDEN CHARGES

When you discuss rates with a prospective home care agency or other provider, make sure to find out about possible hidden charges. For example, there is sometimes a minimum charge per visit, per week, or per month. There may also be higher rates for night and weekend care, which could mean a significant cost increase if you require such care. So, too, some agencies charge extra for in-home assessments, evaluations and for visits by supervisors. These last are necessary elements of overall home care planning and service, however, and should *not* be charged as "extras."

H. SUPPLEMENTS TO HOME CARE

Along with the growth of home care, a number of free or low-cost programs now provide older people with certain services not offered by most agencies. These programs add to the home care services, keep costs down and often make the difference between being able to stay at home and having to enter a nursing facility. Most of all, many of these services give the person receiving care a break in the routine and give family members some relief from their responsibilities.

1. MEALS-ON-WHEELS

Meals-on-Wheels is perhaps the best known supplement to home care. Although good nutrition is essential to health, many older people begin to neglect their diets when shopping, cooking and cleaning become difficult, or when dietary problems restrict food choices. Meals-on-Wheels brings easily affordable food that is hot, tasty, nutritious and ready-to-eat. It also provides daily, friendly human contact that is a welcome diversion in a long day at home.

Almost all communities now have some kind of low-cost meal delivery system for housebound elders, although in some areas there is a waiting list for this service. Funding for Meals-on-Wheels varies, and the service often depends heavily on volunteers, but all of the programs work essentially the same way. For a very small fee, Meals-on-Wheels delivers a hot, nutritional meal once a day, usually around lunchtime. Often, for a slight extra charge, you can also have a snack or another meal, either cold or easily heated, for later in the day.

2. ADULT DAYCARE AND RESPITE CARE

Adult daycare can be either a supplement to home care or a virtual substitute for it. In general, adult daycare centers operate during daytime work hours and provide a meal, monitoring and companionship for people who need some care but are not seriously ill or disabled. Respite care provides a few hours a week of low-cost or free companionship without any active care services. Daycare centers and respite care are often funded by nonprofit organizations, and the programs that do not provide medical care tend to be less expensive than home care.

ADULT DAYCARE CENTERS

Adult daycare centers provide different levels of medical care and therapy, along with meals, companionship, activities and social services. They offer family care givers who work an alternative to using full-time providers at home. For those receiving the care, they can often make the difference between living at home or entering a nursing facility.

Centers affiliated with a hospital or nursing facility may offer extensive medical care—including administering medications and treatments, monitoring specific conditions, health testing and preventive screening—all in keeping with a written, regularly revised health care plan. Rehabilitative therapies should also be available. A physician should be on call and an RN or nurse practitioner available at all times. At centers run by community or public service organizations, less comprehensive medical care may be available.

Participants in adult daycare may stay for a half or full day, one to five days a week; regular, scheduled attendance may be required. Costs depend on the range of services offered and the nature of the sponsoring organization. Many charge according to the ability to pay. If transportation is not provided by the center, the center will often arrange for it.

In addition to medical services, adult daycare centers provide meals and snacks, personal care assistance, exercise, recreation and outings and social and educational programs. Also, social services, including referrals to other agencies and programs, are usually available. Above all, adult daycare centers offer companionship for elders who might otherwise be housebound.

■ _____

FINDING ADULT DAYCARE

If you have difficulty finding an adequate adult daycare center, to get a referral and references for a center nearby contact:

National Institute on Adult Daycare
600 Maryland Avenue, SW, West Wing 100
Washington, DC 20024
(202) 479-1200

RESPITE CARE

Like adult daycare, respite care serves as a break in routine for both those who give and those who receive care. Unlike adult daycare centers, however, respite care does not involve organized activities or services. It provides companionship and monitoring, often by volunteers, for short periods of time on a regular or occasional basis—a few times a week, one weekend a month, or for a full weekend or week when primary care givers are unavailable. Respite care can be provided at home (yours or the care giver's), at a church or community center, or in a nursing facility. It is often sponsored by a community organization and, unless it is at a medical facility, is usually low-cost or even free.

3. SENIOR CENTERS

Most senior centers provide free social and recreational activities, education, information and exercise programs and a hot meal on a drop-in basis to physically self-sufficient elders. Generally, there is no fixed schedule required for participation, although meals and some programs may have to be signed-up for in advance.

While senior centers do not offer personal assistance care, they do provide some respite care, nutrition, organized activities and informal companionship for an elder who does not need monitoring. Senior centers often arrange for transportation to and from the center and sometimes organize outings to places of interest. They are excellent sources of information about services available to seniors, particularly about the individual, independent care givers who can be reliable and less expensive alternatives to agency care but who are sometimes difficult to find.

4. COUNTY HEALTH SCREENING

One of the functions of skilled home health care is to monitor the health of the elder receiving care. If you require less attentive care, however, you may be missing regular health monitoring and screening. As a supplement to doctor visits, many city or county health clinics regularly offer free or low-cost health screening and testing. These clinics can provide adequate general health monitoring if used as part of an ongoing care plan. The public health nurses at these clinics can help schedule a regular program of screening and testing.

5. FAMILY EDUCATION PROGRAMS

A number of public agencies and community organizations—United Way, Red Cross, Visiting Nurses' Association and many hospitals—offer instruction for elders and their families on various aspects of home health care: personal care assistance, such as bathing and movement techniques; exercise; nutrition for special dietary needs; monitoring health conditions and vital signs. Learning these techniques helps assure the safety and well-being of the elder and permits family members to assist with a wider range of home care—avoiding some of the dependence on professional providers. A family education program can also be a good source of information about other available programs, as well as a chance to share information and experiences with other elders and their families.

6. ADDITIONAL SERVICES

In addition to the programs discussed above, there are other specific services available free or at very low cost which can help lighten the burdens of home care.

You can find services to supplement home care much the same way you find home care itself. (Discussed in Section B.) With supplemental care, however, the referrals are more likely to come from local rather than state or regional agencies, and from volunteer and community organizations rather than from institutions or medical sources. The local senior center is usually an excellent source of information, as is the Senior Referral telephone service listed in the white pages of your phone directory. Geriatric case managers can be particularly helpful in finding the small, independent or little-known extra services not provided by home care agencies.

Some of the supplemental services available in many communities are:

SENIOR ESCORT SERVICE

Some people can get around on their own, or with minimum assistance, for short trips to the store or the bank or the park, for example, but are concerned about their safety on the streets. Escort services provide someone to accompany you on short trips; they're often available on fairly short notice.

TRANSPORTATION SERVICE

Many people would make trips to a senior center, the library, a park, or to organized activities if only they had the transportation. There are a number of public agencies and community groups that provide free transportation, often with wheelchair access.

COMPANION SERVICE

Similar to respite care, a companion service can send someone for a few hours a week on a regular schedule, to provide company but not care. The occasional company and conversation of someone who brings good cheer can be a wonderful diversion. These services are mostly volunteer-staffed and community-funded, so there is usually no charge for using them.

HOUSEKEEPING AND GROCERY SERVICES

Many state and local government Departments of Social Services or volunteer programs offer grocery shoppers and part-time housekeepers to do occasional work for low-income physically disabled or impaired elders. When available, these housekeeping and grocery services are offered free or at a very low cost.

TELEPHONE SAFETY SERVICE

Particularly valuable for people who live alone and who do not have family in the vicinity, telephone reassurance programs provide a daily call, at the same time each day, to make sure an elder at home is doing all right. And besides being a safety check, it is always nice to have a brief conversation with someone during the day.

A related service, called Lifeline, is available in many places and provides a telephone emergency response service usually connected directly to a hospital or other emergency health facility. The line can be connected to your phone and maintained for a nominal cost.

ORGANIZED ELDER RESIDENCES

ORGANIZED ELDER RESIDENCES

T he facilities discussed in this chapter are the "in-between" organized residences, which combine some of home's comforts and independence with some of the care and security of a nursing facility. Types of residences range from seniors-only apartments and retirement communities for relatively independent elders, to board and care facilities for people who need more daily assistance. These facilities offer care that either supplements or substitutes for home care, while providing the protected environments but not the medical attention of nursing facilities. Residence can be temporary—while recovering from a serious illness or waiting for full home care arrangements to be made—but most facilities accept only permanent residents.

A Note About Money: One of the first things to realize about residential alternatives is that, in general, they are not cheap.[1] The next thing to know is that, with the exception of some personal care facilities partially covered by Medicaid, there is virtually no coverage by Medicare, Medicaid or private insurance. In other words, you pay all the bills. Nonetheless, with a few exceptions, these residential alternatives are still usually less expensive than nursing facilities and worth considering if home care is not possible but nursing facility care is not needed.

---

[1]The exceptions are subsidized senior housing or congregate housing, discussed later in this chapter, which may charge rent or services on a sliding scale based on income.

■
_____

HOW TO FIND RESIDENTIAL FACILITIES

■ American Association of Homes for the Aging, 1129 20th Street, NW, Washington, DC 20036, can provide you with information about its member housing and residential facilities in your area.

■ Your local Area Agency on Aging provides information about housing and residential facilities. Addresses and phone numbers for Area Agencies can be found in the Resource Directory in the Appendix.

■ The Senior Referral and Information service found in the white pages of the telephone directory can refer you to local residential facilities.

■ Your church, synagogue or ethnic or fraternal organization is often a good source for information about senior housing.

■ Don't forget friends, neighbors, relatives.

A. SENIOR HOUSING

Senior housing, also called congregate or sheltered housing, refers to residential housing complexes built or renovated exclusively for basically independent older people. It provides permanent housing rather than personal care or medical assistance and is designed to make living easier for elders—including elevators, ramps rather than stairs, extra lighting, hand railings and added security. Generally, it offers few services, although many have common social areas and a common dining area where one low-cost meal a day is served. Residents can receive home health care and other services from outside agencies or independent providers.

Many senior housing complexes are subsidized by the federal government or local funding, so rents are lower than on the open market. Rents are sometimes based on income, so that low-income seniors can live in an apartment they would not otherwise be able to afford.

A number of congregate or sheltered apartment complexes, although primarily rental residences, do offer some low-cost extra personal care services within the complex. These may include housekeeping, meals in a common dining room, transportation and shopping services, and exercise, recreation and social activities. Fees for these are billed in addition to rent.

B. RETIREMENT COMMUNITIES

Like senior apartment housing, retirement communities are for independent living. They provide housing rather than personal care and assistance. Many people move into retirement communities merely to escape from the hassles of home ownership and to enjoy the ready-made community of people their own age.

Retirement communities include urban apartment complexes and apartments, townhouses and clusters of individual homes in the suburbs or the country. The major difference between retirement communities and senior housing is that usually one must buy into a retirement community. Like any other residence, the cost depends on size, quality and location—and also on the range of extra services offered. There is often an entrance fee in addition to the cost of the individual living unit.

Retirement communities offer services such as housekeeping, cleaning and maintenance, and sometimes serve meals in a common dining area. Communities may have limited health services on call or on a regular visiting basis, almost always at an extra cost. Many retirement communities provide common social areas, offer adult education classes and transportation to shopping and plan social and recreational activities.

Although you generally purchase and own your residence, ownership may be different than with a regular home. There may be restrictions on the circumstances under which you can sell it or leave it to your heirs. There may also be limits on the sale price, on whom you can sell it to, on how long you must keep it before selling it or on what your heirs are allowed to do with it. Before buying into any retirement community, check the restrictions placed on your property ownership rights.

C. PERSONAL CARE RESIDENCE FACILITIES

Personal care residence facilities are an alternative for people who need a bit more personal assistance than is offered in senior housing or retirement communities, but not as much as is provided in a nursing facility. Most personal care facilities consist of rooms in a larger facility rather than separate apartments, and offer meals and personal care rather than just housing. Some also offer rooms with small kitchens. Personal care residence facilities also typically offer some medical services, although these vary greatly and are generally much less comprehensive than in nursing facilities. Another difference from senior housing or retirement communities is that temporary residence is permitted.

Costs in a personal care facility tend to be somewhat less than in a nursing facility. But because they are not truly nursing facilities, a stay in a personal care facility does not normally qualify for Medicare or private insurance coverage. Medicaid, however, may cover some care for eligible residents. (See Chapter 6 for more information on Medicaid coverage.)

■
_____

I M P O R T A N T

For a complete discussion of what to look for in a personal care facility, see Chapter 4, Nursing Facilities. Except for health care, most things that apply to choosing a nursing facility also apply to a personal care facility.

Although several types of personal care facilities are discussed below, the dividing lines among them are not clearcut. What a facility calls itself does not readily indicate what services it offers. That is something you must determine before entering any residence facility. Do not simply rely on a facility's title.

1. RESIDENTIAL CARE
(BOARD AND CARE) FACILITIES

Board and care or residential care facilities provide a furnished room, all meals, housekeeping and cleaning, varied levels of personal care and assistance, some recreation and transportation, security and resident monitoring. They do *not* provide any medical, nursing or rehabilitation care. For this reason, they tend to feel less hospital-like than many nursing facilities. They are often smaller and more personal and may cost somewhat less than nursing facilities. Charges are generally on a weekly or monthly basis and most have no separate entrance fee.

Note: Depending on level of care and on certification, Medicaid sometimes covers part of the cost of a residential care facility. (See Chapter 6.)

There are virtually no government guidelines or monitoring of residential care facilities, and the amount and quality of personal care varies greatly. It is therefore very important to thoroughly investigate both the level and quality of personal care provided.

■ _____

WHAT TO LOOK FOR IN A RESIDENTIAL CARE FACILITY

Spend some time at the facility and while there, try to get answers to some of the following questions. (For a more detailed discussion of things to look for, see Chapter 4 on nursing facilities. With the exception of health care issues, all questions about a nursing facility also apply to a residential care facility.)

- What are the accommodations like? What do the individual or shared rooms look like? Common and visiting areas? How is privacy guaranteed?
- What services are available? How often? Who provides the services—in-house personnel or outsiders, trained or untrained?
- How are the charges calculated? Can you choose to receive certain services and not others, paying only for the ones you receive?

- Does Medicaid pay for any covered services? No matter what the facility tells you, check with the local Medicaid office as well.
- Who are the supervisors and staff? What is their training and what are their duties?
- Who are the other residents? What is their general condition? How are residents selected?
- What security and safety provisions exist?
- How are complaints about staff, services, accommodations or other residents handled? Are there written policies on such matters?
- What are the reasons and notice requirements by which the facility can terminate residency? Make sure you get them in writing.
- Can the facility offer any references from either former residents and their families or public agencies? Does the facility have any formal relationship with any public agency?
- Is there a relationship with a nursing facility or hospital in case your needs change or there is a medical emergency?

2. SHELTERED CARE FACILITIES

Sheltered care facilities should not be confused with sheltered housing, discussed earlier in this chapter. The key difference is between "housing" and "care facility." Sheltered housing is simply a seniors-only apartment complex with some common areas and design features helpful to independent elders. A sheltered care facility, on the other hand, provides a room in a common facility plus personal and some medical care for dependent elders.

In sheltered care facilities, residents are assumed to be dependent on the staff for many of their regular needs. All meals, cleaning and housekeeping, personal care and some minimal health care are regularly provided, and residents are frequently monitored—in some facilities, 24 hours a day. Charges are usually per day or per week for temporary residents, per month for permanent residents. Medicaid may cover some of the care in some facilities. (See Chapter 6 for detailed information about Medicaid.)

3. LIFE CARE FACILITIES

The premise of life care facilities, also called continuing care or multi-level residential communities, is an excellent one: They are residential complexes that provide all levels of personal and medical services, so that it should not become necessary to move to another facility.

Unfortunately, the reality is not so great. Residents must pay a large entrance fee ($50,000 for a small studio; up to $200,000 or more for a two-bedroom apartment), plus large monthly fees ($500 to $2,000 or more) without any guarantees about the facility's continuing financial stability or quality of care.

Before the risks of life care facilities are discussed, here are the positive things they may provide:

- a variety of living arrangements (separate townhouses, apartments, studios), combined with different services and levels of care—housekeeping, personal care, health care including skilled nursing—at varying entrance costs plus monthly fees.
- ability to upgrade personal services and medical care as needed.
- self-contained facilities with housecleaning, organized social and recreational activities, common dining area with meals available, and extra services such as regular transportation to and from the community.

In short, life care promises to care for you in the same facility for life, no matter what your personal or medical needs become, with the exception of hospitalization, based on fees you know in advance.

■
_____

WARNING

The terms of a life care contract are usually so complicated, and the investment so significant, that before buying it is strongly urged that you have a business adviser, lawyer or accountant review all documents, investigate the financial status and reputation of the facility and thoroughly explain the long-range implications to you.

PITFALLS OF LIFE CARE CONTRACTS

Consumer experts have questioned the abilities of some life care facilities to deliver on all their promises. If the operators of the community do not calculate fees and costs properly, or are poor administrators, they may not be able to deliver in the future the quality of care promised. Some life care communities may also try to dazzle you with promises of lifetime comfort and security without disclosing the limits they put on your ability to leave the community and recoup your investment if you are not satisfied with your life there.

WHAT TO LOOK FOR IN A LIFE CARE FACILITY

RESALE OF MEMBERSHIP

What happens if, for any reason, you want to leave a life care community? And what about your investment if you pass away while a resident in the facility? Can your investment pass to your heirs?

Many life care facilities do not permit you to sell your "membership" at all. In these facilities, you do not actually own your apartment. The huge initial downpayment is an entrance fee, not part of a property purchase. Consequently, when you die you leave no legal interest in the property to pass on to your heirs and your investment ends when your residence does. In other words, once the life care operators have your money, it is theirs for good no matter how short your stay.

Other facilities will permit you to sell your membership, or leave it to your heirs, but may put severe restrictions on the value that can be taken out and the terms under which it can be sold. Still other facilities will refund a portion of your entrance fee if you leave the facility within a certain period of time, but they exact a huge penalty—usually one to five per cent of the fee per month for every month you have been a resident.

FEE CONTROL

Are there any hidden charges? Are there controls on fee increases? In addition to the hefty entrance fees, life care facilities charge a large monthly fee and sometimes additional fees for extra services. Some facilities also increase the monthly fees if you must move into a nursing care section of the facility. Before you join a life care facility, find out what these charges are. Even more important, since you may be in the facility for many years, make sure it is clear in your written contract how, when and by how much the facility is permitted to raise each of those charges.

Without written contract limitations on fee increases, the facility may make you pay later for its own poor management. There will certainly be some provision for rate increases based on inflation or rises in the cost of medical care, but these should be strictly controlled in the written contract.

SUFFICIENCY OF MEDICAL CARE

Who is on the medical staff? How much nursing is available? What about personal care aides? What are the skill levels of the people who provide the care? Is Medicare-covered skilled nursing available? What does the nursing care wing of the facility look like? What are the extra health care charges?

In a life care community, part of what you pay for is the facility's promise to provide lifetime personal assistance and medical care. When many people look at life care facilities, however, they concentrate on the living quarters and social activities, rather than at the health care staff, programs and physical facilities. Only when you have fully evaluated the available personal assistance and medical care will you know what you are buying. (To help you make that evaluation, see the checklists in Chapter 4 that pertain to nursing facilities.)

FACILITY'S LONG-TERM FINANCIAL STABILITY

How long has the facility been in operation? Do its financial records indicate that it is on sound financial footing?

Unfortunately, there have been a few cases of life care facilities which were so financially unsound that they were forced to go into bankruptcy or to totally reorganize with different care at higher prices. The residents of these facilities were left either with lower quality care or were forced to pay large additional sums of money to the facility to keep up the level of care.

Any time you buy into a plan for future care, you are taking a gamble that the facility will later be able to deliver the same quality of care it promises when you join. Consider that its ability to provide quality care in the future, without having to raise rates exorbitantly, depends on its long-term financial stability—always a difficult factor to assess accurately.

NURSING FACILITIES

NURSING FACILITIES

Despite an increase in available home care and senior housing, one out of every two women and one of three men over age 65 will enter a nursing facility some time in their lives. The stay may be a long one: 25% of all nursing facility stays last more than a year and many last two years, or more.

PLANNING AND FINANCES

How nursing facility residence is paid for can determine whether or not you can hold onto your life's savings. (See Chapters 6 and 7 for explanations of Medicaid and answers to other nursing facility financial questions.) When possible, financial planning *before* entering a facility can be extremely important.

As soon as you begin to see that current living arrangements may be insufficient in the foreseeable future, begin planning. Many nursing facilities operate at full capacity and may not be able to accept a new resident on short notice. To guarantee getting into the facility of your choice—and in some rural areas, there may be very little choice—make your decisions as early as possible.

Although there are different levels of care in nursing facilities, all involve full-time residence and include room and board, monitoring, personal assistance, nursing and other health care for people who are physically or mentally unable to attend to all their own needs. There is a great range in the levels of care available in what are broadly termed "nursing facilities." Hospital-based skilled nursing facilities provide short-term, intensive medical care and monitoring for people recovering from acute illness or injury. Other facilities—what used to be called "rest homes"—provide long-term room and board and assistance with personal care such as dressing, eating and exercising, but little or no health care.

Although many people prefer to arrange for long-term care outside of nursing facilities, others find comfort and security in the services that nursing facilities offer. Many people would prefer to remain outside a nursing facility but because of their condition, circumstances or the unavailability of in-home services, they can only receive adequate care in a residential nursing facility. Unfortunately, as sometimes makes the news, some facilities exist with substandard living conditions and even dangerous lack of care. Still others give basic care that meets technical health standards but offer little else, and have an atmosphere that is debilitating or demoralizing to the residents.

There are, however, excellent nursing facilities that provide high quality care while assisting residents to maintain active lives with a full measure of dignity. But because there are many levels and types of nursing and personal care, the task is to find a good, affordable facility that is right for you.

■

WHERE TO FIND NURSING FACILITY REFERRALS

Hospital discharge planner. They will often be available for advice if you are going straight from a hospital to a nursing facility.

Your doctor. Ask your doctor about personal experience he or she may have had with area nursing facilities.

Organization focusing on specific illness. Check with organizations that focus on your particular illness or disability, such as the American Heart Association, American Cancer Society, American Diabetes Association, or Alzheimer's Disease Foundation.

National long-term care organizations. A number of private organizations such as American Association of Homes for the Aging specialize in long-term care and give referrals to local facilities. (See the Resource Directory in the Appendix.)

Government agencies. You can often get targeted referrals from the federal area Agencies on Aging, or from state and local agencies found through Senior Referral and

Information numbers in the white pages of the phone book or your local county social services or family services agency.

Church, ethnic or fraternal organizations. Ask about nursing facilities members have used successfully or that are operated by or affiliated with the church or organization.

Relatives, friends and neighbors. They may have had experience with a nursing facility or know someone who has. They are often your best source of information.

A. LEVELS OF MEDICAL CARE

An essential thing to learn about nursing facilities is that levels of care vary even within the same facility, ranging from intensive 24-hour nursing care for the seriously ill, to minimal personal assistance without any active nursing or other medical care. The long-term physical and emotional health of a resident depends on getting the right amount of care, enough but *not too much*.

Many people in nursing facilities are in relatively good physical and mental health but do not have enough family or resources to get assistance at home. A person who needs minimal care and who has the health and energy to remain active is in danger of losing much of that vitality in a facility set up to care for people who are critically ill. The higher the level of care, the more hospital-like some facilities tend to be, and the more ill and frail the residents. Such a setting can quickly drain a healthier resident of energy and spirit.

So, too, the higher the level of care, the higher the cost. Higher-level care may initially be covered by Medicare or private insurance while a lower level is not, but what coverage there is will be very limited. (See Chapters 5 and 6 for a full discussion of what costs are covered by Medicare, Medicaid and private insurance.) And if residence in the high-level facility exceeds Medicare or insurance coverage, it may cost you more than a lower-care facility that you pay for entirely yourself.

■
_____

NOTE

Bear in mind that regardless of what a nursing facility calls itself,
you must carefully investigate the care provided and check *in
advance* with both the facility and with Medicare, Medicaid and
your private insurance carrier to find out the availability and
terms of coverage for your residence in the facility.

1. HOSPITAL-BASED SKILLED NURSING FACILITIES

Hospital-based skilled nursing facilities, also known as extended care
facilities, are departments within hospitals. They provide the highest
levels of medical and nursing care, including 24-hour monitoring and
intensive rehabilitative therapies. They are intended to follow acute
hospital care due to serious illness, injury or surgery.

Unlike other nursing facilities, hospital-based facilities are not for
permanent residence, but for a short term until a patient can be sent home
or maintained elsewhere. Hospital-based facilities are very expensive ($150
to $200 per day), but the average stay is generally almost always for a
matter of weeks only and, for those who qualify, is usually well covered by
Medicare or private insurance. (See Chapters 5 and 10.)

2. SKILLED NURSING FACILITIES

Non-hospital-based skilled nursing facilities (SNFs) provide a relatively
high level of nursing and other medical care, as well as personal care
and assistance, for people whose illnesses or impairments require close
monitoring.

Around-the-clock nursing is available from licensed vocational or
practical nurses, with at least one supervising registered nurse on duty
at all times. In addition to nursing, most other prescribed medical
services can be provided, including various rehabilitative therapies. A
SNF can be for either short-term, post-hospitalization recovery or long-
term residence for serious chronic illness or impairment.

The cost of SNF care ranges from $50 to $150 per day. Medicare
and private insurance will pay only up to their coverage limits, and
only if SNF care has been specifically prescribed by a physician. (See

the rules for SNF coverage by Medicare, Medicaid and private insurance in Chapters 5, 6 and 10.)

3. INTERMEDIATE CARE FACILITIES

Intermediate care facilities (ICFs) provide less nursing and other medical care than SNFs. ICFs are for long-term residents with chronic illness or impairment whose conditions are not as acute as those of SNF residents and who are usually ambulatory.

Staff is geared as much toward personal care and assistance as to medical care, although there is always a licensed vocational or practical nurse on duty. Only basic physical therapy is usually included, although other rehabilitative therapies can be arranged as extra services.

Costs range from $40 to $75 per day. There is no coverage by Medicare and private insurance coverage is rare, probably with prior approval required. Medicaid, however, may cover much of the cost of ICF care. (See Chapter 6.)

■ _____

NOTE

Because they are not able to charge as much as SNFs, and because coverage from outside sources is limited, there are very few facilities that are set up to be ICFs alone. (But see "Multi-Level Facilities," Section 4, below.)

4. MULTI-LEVEL FACILITIES

Care needs change over time. But once someone is comfortable in a particular facility, it can be very disturbing to move to another facility if greater care is required. It most often makes sense, then, to choose a nursing facility that offers more than one level of care.

Some hospital-based skilled nursing facilities have intermediate care facilities attached. Someone going directly from the hospital into short-term intensive monitoring and care can receive it in the skilled care section and remain in the same facility, with the same staff, when his or her condition improves. Similarly, it is common for non-hospital facilities to combine skilled with intermediate or personal care, permitting those recovering from serious conditions to move from skilled to lower care when their condition improves, or long-term residents to move to skilled care if their condition worsens.

Although a multi-level facility offers flexibility, if a facility is too diversified, the personalized attention so important to a long-term resident can suffer. This is particularly true if a facility concentrates too much on its high-skill medical care and neglects the individualized non-medical care and assistance that long-term residents need most. In addition, the high cost of skilled medical care may be passed on to long-term residents who do not use it. So, be wary if your tours of a facility and conversations with its administrators focus entirely on shiny, high-technology medical equipment.

Finally, pay careful attention to how payments are required to be made at a multi-level facility. Initial Medicare or private insurance coverage for skilled nursing care does *not* mean coverage will continue after care switches to a non-skilled level. Always check with the facility, with Medicare, with your private insurance carrier and with Medicaid *before* entering a multi-level facility—before entering any kind of facility—to see which levels of care will be covered and under what terms and conditions.

■
_____

WARNING: "LIFE CARE" CONTRACTS

Some multi-level care facilities offer what are called life care contracts. These usually involve paying a large, non-refundable fee, and sometimes also transferring assets to the facility, in exchange for its promise to care for the resident for life.

Life care contracts may provide a false sense of security and tend to be bad risks for a number of reasons. If the facility runs into financial trouble, you may be out of luck. Once you have paid all your money, there is little incentive left for it to provide good care.

And once you've put all your eggs in that facility's basket, you will have few choices if you are not happy there, or if it cannot handle your care. Also, the amount of money you pay may be well out of proportion to the length of your residence. For these reasons and more, if you are offered a life care contract, *proceed with extreme caution*. For a detailed discussion of life care arrangements, see Life Care Facilities in Chapter 3.

B. CHOOSING THE RIGHT FACILITY

Once you have determined which facilities in your area are affordable and provide the appropriate general level of care, you must decide which one best suits your needs and preferences.

The experts to turn to for guidance are the residents themselves. Most nursing facility residents, studies have shown, care very little about high-tech medical gear, or even about medical care. Rather, their most important concerns involve their ability to maintain some independence, to participate in decisions about daily life and to retain contact with the outside world.

Because so many of these and other concerns discussed below cannot be guaranteed in writing or demonstrated in a quick tour, it is important to spend as much time as possible at a facility before making a decision to receive care there. Make separate visits during the day, evening and night, and during one or more meals. And to the extent possible, talk with current residents and their families.

1. OWNERSHIP AND MANAGEMENT

The management and hands-on care personnel determine the quality of daily life in a nursing facility. Who actually owns it normally has little to do with the quality of care you'll find there.

FOR-PROFIT FACILITIES

About three-fourths of all nursing facilities are operated for profit, many of them owned by big corporations. There is a popular but not necessarily accurate belief that in profit-making facilities, the dominating desire to make money means skimping on patient care. Research has shown that this is *not* usually the case. Profit-making facilities may be better managed than nonprofit ones and therefore deliver better care for the dollar. Similarly, studies have found that keeping patients satisfied is important to for-profit facilities because their economic health depends on keeping their beds filled.

NONPROFIT FACILITIES

The flip-side of negative beliefs about profit-making facilities is the notion that those run by nonprofit philanthropic, charitable or religious organizations will provide quality care because their only interest is to "do good" for residents. But nonprofit organizations often give no more than their name and tax advantage to a nursing facility while its everyday management is handled by people who only work under contract with the organization. Even when the nonprofit organization takes an active role in running the facility—usually several facilities— there is no guarantee it will be any better at the job than profit-making managers. The test of care quality comes on the floor of the facility itself and not in the boardrooms of its owners.

GROUP AFFILIATION

Many nursing facilities are operated by or affiliated with religious, ethnic or fraternal organizations. Depending both on your interest and on the degree to which the affiliation affects daily life in the facility, this can be either good or bad. A particular affiliation may mean you and the other residents will have similar backgrounds and interests which can make for a real feeling of community. Also, there may be specially-targeted activities at the facility in which you will enjoy participating.

On the other hand, if a group or organization to which you do not belong dominates the social activity of a facility, it may make you an outsider and may also limit the availability of other, non-sectarian activities. Be aware of a facility's affiliation and its influence on daily life there.

2. COST

A popular idea about a purchase of any kind is that you get what you pay for—and the more something costs, the better the quality.

With nursing facilities, high price often means sophisticated and expensive medical equipment and staff. And although most residents will never need them, every resident winds up paying. Similarly, some facilities are expensive because they have a shiny new building to pay for.

Many smaller, less expensive facilities with less high-tech equipment can provide a more comfortable setting with more individual attention and participation for residents. Of course, you must

make certain that lower cost does not reflect a lack of essential services
or of qualified personnel. But these are things to investigate and cannot
be assumed from the cost of the care alone.

■

MORE IS NOT LESS

While one might guess that larger facilities cost less because
they operate on an economy of scale, in general it is just the
opposite. On the average, larger facilities cost more to operate
than smaller ones, probably because of more and higher-level
medical services and larger administrative staffs.

3. THE FACILITY

LOCATION

For a number of reasons, where a facility is located can be extremely
significant. Continuing contact with people and life outside the facility
is of the residents' greatest concerns, and location can affect that
contact in a number of ways.

Visiting: Can friends and relatives get there easily? Is it near
public transportation? The ease with which people can visit has a direct
bearing on how often they do.

Outings: Are there places nearby—a park, library, senior
center—where elders can be taken for outings, either by visitors or by
staff?

Immediate surroundings: Is the surrounding area noisy,
peaceful, ugly, safe? What can be seen and heard through the windows
during the day and night? Are short walks or a bit of lounging outside
possible?

NUMBER OF BEDS AND RESIDENTS

As with most questions about nursing facilities, there is no simple
guideline about whether a large or small one is best. It is mostly a
matter of your own needs and tastes, and of the quality of care
delivered. Of concern when assessing large facilities, those with over
100 beds, is whether their size means they're too institutional, too

cold—and whether they still provide personal attention and permit residents to participate in their own care.

A small facility, on the other hand, may not have all the services and skilled personnel such as dieticians, rehabilitative therapists, and social workers, that a larger one has. But smaller facilities tend to be more personal and homey and allow residents greater control over their own daily lives.

THE FACILITY'S "FEEL"

What is your first impression when you walk through the door? It may be the same general impression, conscious or unconscious, that a resident has all the time.

Homeyness: A facility should be as unlike a hospital as is consistent with good health care. It should be colorful, with personal, individual touches on walls and tables. Some facilities encourage residents to decorate their rooms and common areas; others have regulations against it. There should also be plenty of light, both from windows and lamps.

Healthfulness: The facility should be clean and free from strong odors. Infections and viruses pass easily in group living situations, and they can be very serious for elders. The space should not feel cramped; crowding is both physically and psychologically unhealthy. And the air should not be too hot, too cold, or too stuffy.

■
_____

FACILITY HEALTH INSPECTIONS

Nursing facility health conditions are periodically inspected by the state. Each facility should have on file its most recent state or federal inspection report, called a Statement of Deficiencies & Plan of Correction. This report is *not* confidential and should be made available to you on request. Even the best facility is likely to have some minor complaints against it, but the report can also give you an idea of whether there are any serious problems.

PUBLIC AREAS

Prospective residents often pay much less attention to common rooms than to residents' private rooms. But the comfort and attraction of the public areas affect the amount of time a resident spends out of his or her room, out of bed, and so may have a bearing on how active the resident remains. The following are some of the things you might consider.

A "quiet" room: Although one advantage of a nursing facility is that residents do not spend too much time alone, it can also be a problem. Most residents share rooms, and privacy can sometimes be difficult to find. It's important that some room or area is available for solitude or at least quiet—where there is no radio, television or group activities and where it is understood that people are to be left to themselves.

Eating areas: Food and rules about eating are discussed more fully below, but you should spend time both where food is served and eaten—dining room, private rooms, other areas of the facility—while residents are actually eating and, if possible, eat a meal there with the residents.

Social, TV and activity rooms: While television can be good company for facility residents, it can also become a real annoyance. If there are televisions in all common areas, and they are always on, that can interfere with other activities, such as having a simple conversation. Whether or not there is a "quiet" room, it should be possible to socialize somewhere without a TV blaring.

The social and activity rooms should be clean and comfortable and should have some personal touches. A simple way to tell whether the residents find these common rooms inviting is to see how many people are using them.

Outside areas: Is there a courtyard or other outside area where residents can spend time? Is there a garden in which residents can work? Both the air and change of scene from inside can be very refreshing to residents.

Visiting areas: Is there a place other than the resident's room for private visits? Must visiting take place in a room used for other purposes as well? Does the facility encourage visiting or make it seem like a bother?

RESIDENTS' PRIVATE ROOMS

Many people who enter a nursing facility have not shared a room with anyone else for a long time, yet virtually all nursing facilities provide only double or triple rooms. Adjusting to the loss of privacy and need for compromise that go with sharing a bedroom can be difficult. The set-up and rules of the facility can make this transition either easier or harder. The following list suggests some things to look for:

Size: Are there single rooms, double, or triple? Are there adjoining bathrooms? Are the bathrooms set up to ensure privacy?

Light: Is there a window that lets in natural light? Are there individual reading lights near each bed? Can the lights be used without disturbing a roommate's sleep?

Structure: Does the set-up of the room, furniture and perhaps a curtain between beds allow some privacy for each roommate? Is there someplace to sit other than on the bed? Are there places for visitors to sit and visit privately? Can furnishings be moved around?

Security: Theft is a common problem in nursing facilities. Is there a place where personal possessions can be kept safely and easily retrieved? Is there a call button within reach of each bed that connects to the central aide station and can only be turned off at the bed?

Comfort: Is private furniture allowed in the room? Is room temperature controlled by each room? Are telephones, radios or televisions permitted in the rooms? If so, what are the rules to protect roommates from too much noise?

4. SERVICES AND ACTIVITIES

Nursing facilities do not all offer the same services and activities beyond basic personal and medical care. Some facilities focus on exercise and therapy for physical impairments, others on social or educational programs, still others on developing residents' independence and memory. It is important to match services and activities with needs. For example, if a resident does not have the physical or mental capacity to be very active, recreational and social programs may be much less important than the amount of personal staff attention to cleanliness and comfort. For more active residents, though, activities that encourage independent thought and movement may be crucial to maintaining the highest possible levels of health.

Matching services and activities with needs cannot be done entirely in advance because it's difficult to anticipate what needs will be most important. Also, needs change over time. Try to choose a facility that encourages resident input into services and activities, and is attentive to a resident's individual needs. Discuss the flexibility of services and activities with the staff and listen for indications that residents' dignity, independence and individual differences are important.

REHABILITATION THERAPY

Is the particular physical, respiratory, speech or other therapy you need regularly available in the facility or must special arrangements be made? Does the resident have to go outside the facility to receive the therapy? Is there extra cost?

SOCIAL ACTIVITIES AND OTHER SERVICES

The greatest concern of many nursing facility residents is for contact with the outside world—seeing family and other visitors, physically leaving the facility, receiving news, phone calls and mail.

Outings: Does the facility regularly organize outings to places and activities such as the library, park, local senior center, shopping? Is transportation provided? Are escorts available for a simple walk?

Incoming activity: Are visiting speakers and activities scheduled regularly? Is there a program of outside volunteers who participate with residents in some program or activity?

Organized events: Look at the facility's weekly or monthly calendar of events. Is there stimulation for mind and body—education, information and exercise—as well as just entertainment? Do organized activities take place in the evening as well as the day? Do people from outside the facility participate?

Personal care: Are there services for personal grooming and cleanliness, such as a visiting barber or hairdresser and a way to have clothes washed and cleaned? Does a dentist or dental hygienist visit the facility?

Social service assistance: Is there a counselor or social worker who can assist with family problems, paperwork, financial organization and referrals for outside services?

FACILITY-WIDE RULES

Every facility has rules by which all residents and visitors must abide.
Do they seem reasonable? Do the administrators seem willing to be
flexible with those rules to meet individual needs? Ask to see the
written rules and also try to find out about important rules of daily life
which are not listed.

Visiting: When and where is visiting allowed? Are there any
particular rules about children? What about phone calls in and out? Can
visitors eat facility meals with residents?

Meals: Are mealtimes flexible? If a meal is missed, is there
other food available to eat? Must meals be eaten in the dining area? Is
food from outside the facility allowed?

Hours: Is there a set time when all patients are awakened? Is
there a rule about having to get dressed? About going to bed? Watching
television? Lights out? Is there a curfew for residents who have gone on
an outing?

Bathing: If a resident needs assistance bathing, does he or she
retain a reasonable choice about when and how often?

Smoking and drinking: What are the rules about
smoking? Are there separate areas for smokers? Is alcohol allowed at
all, and if so, how is it monitored?

Privacy: Can a resident keep the private room door closed at
will, or only during night hours? Must staff knock before entering? Is
there privacy in the bathroom?

Privately-hired aides: Some facilities allow residents to
supplement the personal care staff with privately-hired aides. This
flexibility may be a good thing, but be wary if the practice is common.
It may mean the staff relies on the outside aides and gives less care and
personal attention to residents.

MEDICATION CONTROL

Over-medication is a serious problem for many older people—
particularly for nursing facility residents. If several different medications
are required, keeping track of them is sometimes difficult.

Some nursing facilities also encourage residents to take "as-
needed" medication—sedatives, relaxants, sleeping medicines—instead
of responding to their needs. It is important to note whether a facility
monitors residents' medication carefully. The facility should:

- keep a written record for the personal physician and family to review;
- have a policy of periodic review of all medications a resident is taking;
- have a policy that any new medication shall be cleared in writing with a responsible family member; and
- have a clearly-stated rule about the residents' right to refuse unwanted medication.

■

SPECIAL WARNING ON DRUG USE

Some nursing facilities prescribe and administer *psychotropic drugs*, also known as "chemical straight jackets." These drugs make residents easy for the facility to care for because, in essence, they turn active residents into zombies. Not only do these drugs rob residents of their humanity while they're directly under the influence, but they can do lasting physical and emotional damage as well.

Any good nursing facility should be willing to show you its written policy on psychotropic drugs. The policy should specify that no such drugs can be administered to a resident without the *written* consent of either the resident or certain designated family members, that any such written consent be for a limited period of time and that the designated family members and the resident's physician be notified of the administration of any such drugs.

Similarly, many nursing facilities frequently use restraints to hold a resident into a bed or chair. Although in some limited circumstances restraints may be necessary for people who are in danger of falling if left unattended, restraints may be used like psychoactive drugs merely to "manage" residents who require more attention than the facility wants to give. Make sure to find out what the facility's policy is on the use of restraints. It should be clearly stated, should permit restraints only when the resident presents an immediate danger of physical injury to himself or herself or to others, and should require that a designated family member be notified when restraints are to be used.

MEDICAL RECORDS

Although technically required to keep records only of certain medical and nursing procedures they provide, a thorough nursing facility will also keep a written record of a resident's medical condition and of outside treatment by doctors, clinics and hospitals. It can be very helpful to a resident and to his or her physician if the facility keeps a written record of health problems that have not warranted medical treatment but have affected the resident's comfort and well-being— such as problems with elimination, digestion or sleeping, depression, too much time in bed, bedsores.

5. OTHER RESIDENTS

When considering a nursing facility, try to make several visits there and speak to some of the residents as you consider the matters discussed below.

SIMILAR LEVELS OF CARE

Small facilities should admit only residents with relatively similar care needs; large facilities should provide only one level of care in each separate area or wing. There are several reasons for this. First, when care is kept to one level, personnel can be specialized; they may be better at what they do if they have fewer things to do. Costs may also be kept down because residents aren't paying for services they don't need.

There are also less tangible reasons for wanting to be with people whose needs are similar to your own. Residents can share their concerns and their ways of coping with common problems. Also, they need not be confronted daily with problems much different or more severe than their own. This is particularly important where mental orientation or capacity is concerned.

ROOM ASSIGNMENT

Most nursing facilities have two or three beds per room. In surveys of residents, roommate selection ranks right behind contact with friends and relatives as most important.

Some people prefer to have a roommate in similar physical condition so that they can better understand each other's needs and concerns. Other people do not mind having a roommate with greater needs; it allows them to be of help. Still others would prefer a roommate in better physical condition so that they can receive extra help. Whatever your preference, find out whether the facility will take it into account in assigning a roommate.

There is also the matter of finding someone with common interests, religious or ethnic background, language and habits—smoking or late nights, for example. Will the facility consider these things when assigning a roommate? If so, make sure to let them know the things that are most important to you.

RESIDENTS' CONDITION AND ACTIVITY

You can tell a lot about a nursing facility simply by walking around and looking carefully at the residents. Are most extremely ill or disabled? Do people appear comfortable? Are they reasonably neat and clean? Do you see smiles, hear friendly conversation among residents and between residents and staff? Are residents moving about the facility and being active in some way, or are they mostly in their rooms?

By checking the common areas, you can tell whether the residents are doing things together or only on their own. It may take several visits, at different times of the day, to get a feel for this. Are there any ongoing communal activities, such as a newsletter, a garden, regular outings, some volunteer project? Be sure to ask.

6. PERSONNEL

As with judgments about residents, getting a sense of the staff requires spending some time at the facility during a normal day's activities.

PERSONAL CARE AIDES

In virtually every nursing facility, 90% of direct resident care is provided by personal care aides—also called assistants, attendants or orderlies. These are the foot soldiers of nursing facility care, and their competence and attitude are most important to the health and well-being of residents. There are several things to find out them.

Numbers: Does it seem that there are enough aides for the number of residents? Are there residents who seem to want attention from an aide but are not receiving it?

Turnover: How long have people worked at the facility? Long-term employment generally means that both aides and residents are satisfied with the aides' work. A rapid turnover of aides may be a bad sign, although even the best facilities sometimes have a hard time keeping staff.

Language: If English is not the first language of the resident, how many people on the staff speak the resident's first language? The reverse may also be true: What percentage of the staff speaks understandable English?

Intangibles: The importance of the courtesy, friendliness and efficiency of the personal care aides to both residents and visitors cannot be overemphasized. But the only way to judge this is to see the aides and residents in their daily interchanges. Is there easy conversation? Do the aides seem to pay attention to what the residents want? Do the aides have a neat and professional appearance?

Remember, as with any group of people, not every aide and every resident are going to get along. The crucial thing is not that every interaction is smiling and efficient, but that most contacts are cordial and responsive to a resident's needs.

AVAILABLE PROFESSIONAL STAFF

The number of personnel listed on stationery with impressive certificates and licenses matters very little. What counts is how much time any of them actually spends with residents. How often does the facility's physician check on medical care standards? How often do licensed nurses make rounds? How easy is it to schedule a rehabilitation therapist? How much hands-on care do the professional level personnel provide and how much are they just supervising? To what extent can a resident request direct care from one of the professional staff?

Direct physician care will almost always come from your own doctor rather than the facility's doctors, so it is important to find out what limits are placed on your doctor's visits to you. You also need to know your doctor's policy about nursing facility visits in general, as well as his or her ability to get to the facility you are considering.

OUTSIDE HELP

Find out whether the facility permits or arranges for extra outside help.

Volunteers: Many facilities make good use of volunteers from public service agencies and programs. Some simply provide extra personal attention or companionship, while others bring special educational skills or social programs. These volunteers are a good link to the outside world and give residents a change of pace and face from the regular staff.

Private aid: Does the facility allow part-time private assistance of any sort from outside the facility, such as a private duty care assistant, chiropractor, massage therapist or private duty nurse?

7. FOOD

In a nursing facility, the importance of meals goes beyond merely getting the right nutrients. Meals are central activities in a resident's day—a social event and a source of pleasure when many other events and pleasures are no longer available. In inquiring about a facility's food service, don't restrict yourself to looking at a menu or seeing that a dietician is an official member of the staff. Instead, *visit the facility's dining areas during one or more meals, and eat the food with residents.* There are several things to ask, look and taste for.

Tastiness: Simple truths are often overlooked, such as the fact that the nutritional value of food is wasted if the food is not eaten. Another is that if food tastes lousy, people eat less of it. Freshness and variety also help keep people interested. Check menus from a week or two and see how often fresh foods are served and how often dishes are repeated.

Preferences and restrictions: No group living facility can cater to the different food whims and desires of all its residents. But residents should be offered some choice in meals, and the facility should respond to strong likes and dislikes. Dietary restrictions, whether for health, digestive or religious reasons, must be strictly followed. The facility should keep a *written* record of any such restriction for each resident, and the kitchen staff should consult it before, not after, planning and preparing meals.

Extra food: Not everyone's appetite runs by the standard meal clock. Some people prefer, or need, to eat a little bit several times a day. Other people who are up at "odd" hours get hungry. And many people get pleasure from special foods made by friends or relatives or a favorite neighborhood bakery. A facility that is too rigid about food is not taking care of important needs.

Does the facility serve snacks, tea or coffee between meals, or at least make such things available to residents? Do the snacks include fresh fruit and other healthful foods? Can residents eat the snacks where and when they want—particularly, in their own rooms—or only at designated times and places?

Dining area: The first thing to pay attention to when you visit the dining area during a meal is whether the residents are eating the food. That will tell you a lot. Observe whether the staff is helpful with residents who need assistance eating. Are residents comfortable and is the area clean? Ask if dining times are flexible. Do residents have enough time with their meal or is food rushed in and out?

8. FAMILY INVOLVEMENT

Although one benefit of a nursing facility is its ready-made community of companions and helpers, there are important benefits in active family involvement in the resident's life. Residents rate personal contact—by visits, phone, mail and outings—at the top of their list of concerns. And no matter how good a facility's own outreach programs are, a resident's ability to stay in touch with the larger community requires help from friends and relatives.

Whether family and friends are actively involved in a resident's life depends to no small degree on whether the facility encourages their participation. Families should be regularly invited to participate in activities with residents. Visiting should be encouraged rather than merely tolerated. Therefore, there should be adequate space, comfort and privacy in visiting areas and wide and flexible visiting hours. Visiting should be permitted during meals and there should be wide latitude in taking residents for outings.

Together, the staff and resident's family should regularly review the resident's condition and care. Find out what the procedures are for family consultation about problems or changes in the resident's care plan or room or roommate assignment. Another thing to ask about is whether there is an organized family support group or network which keeps residents' families in touch with one another.

9. DECISION-MAKING

Residents' long-term health and comfort directly depend on a facility's procedures for making decisions about their care. A good facility should have standardized procedures about residents' daily care decisions. Review them before deciding about a particular facility.

RESIDENTS' PROBLEMS AND COMPLAINTS

It is a sad but widely-recognized truth that there is significant patient abuse and neglect in nursing facilities. And there are also many smaller problems that, if unattended, can make a resident's life miserable. It is therefore very important that there are specific procedures for residents and family members to lodge a complaint or discuss a problem about a particular staff person, a method or type of care, or a facility rule or condition.

The danger of not having an explicit complaint procedure is that a resident will not know with whom to speak, or will get a run-around from staff members who claim they have no authority to do anything to right the wrong. Find out how complaints are handled and make certain that the process guarantees a response from an identifiable person in authority.[1]

Similarly, there should be a regular procedure to register a complaint or discuss a problem about a roommate or other resident. Find out what these procedures are, and what needs to be done to make a room change at the resident's request.

---

[1]If a facility refuses to respond to a resident's complaints, there are state and local government agencies which can step in. See the discussion of the Nursing Facility Ombudsman, below.

FACILITY-IMPOSED CHANGES

For financial and other reasons, when there are vacancies in double rooms, a facility may want to move residents around. Or, because of a change in a resident's condition that requires a different level of care, the facility may believe a room change is necessary. However, the resident may disagree. It is therefore important that a resident have a right to be notified in advance of a change, and that the facility have rules that limit the circumstances under which such changes can be made.

As with a room change, the facility may decide that the particular non-medical care a resident has been receiving is no longer necessary, or that new types of costlier or more restrictive care are required. Find out how these decisions are made and what rights the resident has regarding them. Also make sure there is a provision for consultation and notification of the family.

For all decisions about medical care or changes in condition, specific written procedures should be set out, including:

- what decisions can be made by aides and what must be decided by the nurse on duty;
- when the facility's attending physician must be consulted about a change in medical care or condition;
- when the resident's personal physician must be consulted about a change in condition or a possible change in care;
- when the resident's family must be notified of a change in care or condition.

NURSING FACILITY OMBUDSMAN

The federal government funds a program, administered by each state's Agency on Aging, which makes available to nursing facility residents an ombudsman—a kind of trouble-shooter to mediate unresolved problems between residents or their families and a nursing facility. State and local governments also frequently have a nursing facility ombudsman available. If the ombudsman cannot bring the two sides to an agreement, he or she has the authority to take action to curb nursing facility abuses. There is no charge to the resident for the services of the ombudsman.

You can find your local ombudsman by looking in the white pages of the telephone book under Ombudsman, Long-Term Care Ombudsman or Nursing Facility Ombudsman. If you cannot find a local number, call the state office of the ombudsman program. (The address and phone number for each state office is in the Resource Directory in the Appendix of this book.) Or consult the local Senior Referral and Information listed in the white pages of the telephone directory.

C. ENTERING A FORMAL RESIDENCE CONTRACT

All facilities have a formal written document which both you and a facility representative sign. It does not matter whether this document is called a "contract" or an "agreement" or something similar. What does matter is that all important terms and conditions of residence and care are included, so that both you and the facility are clear about them. If you are unsure of any terms and conditions, consider having an attorney or someone else familiar with nursing facility care review it with you before signing. Even if you do not consult with anyone else, take the agreement home and review it carefully before signing.

If something important to you is not included in the facility's pre-printed agreement, discuss it with the proper facility official, and when you've reached an agreement, write it on a separate piece of paper, signed and dated by both you and the facility official and attach it to the rest of the agreement.

■

NOTE ON MEDICARE AND MEDICAID

Have the facility put in writing how much of these fees it believes are covered by Medicare and Medicaid. (For a full discussion of Medicare and Medicaid coverage, see Chapters 5 and 6.) Whatever the facility tells you, also check directly with the local Medicare and Medicaid offices.

1. WHAT TO LOOK FOR IN A WRITTEN AGREEMENT

The agreement should spell out the specific health care, personal care, equipment and supplies included in the level of care for which you are paying a regular daily, weekly or monthly fee. This should include frequency of nursing care and physical or other therapies, plus number of meals and special dietary needs.

Room: The agreement should specify the number of beds in the resident's room, as well as any other features that distinguish the type of room from others in the facility and are important to you—such as the room size, bathroom facilities, windows, location in the building.

Extra charges and adjustments: The agreement should specify what services, equipment and supplies are charged as extra—above the regular rate. The agreement should also specify amounts to be subtracted for such things as meals eaten outside of the facility and time spent away, such as vacations or time in the hospital.

Some contracts require that residents purchase their medications at the facility's own pharmacy. Since the rates there may be considerably higher than at outside pharmacies, this is in effect a forced extra charge. Find out in advance whether this is the policy at any facility you are considering.

Rate changes: The agreement should spell out whether, and how much, the regular rate will go up or down if the level of care is changed, whether the regular rate is guaranteed to remain the same for any length of time and how much notice must be given before rates are raised.

Change in funding: As discussed in Chapter 5, Medicare and private insurance coverage for nursing facility care is very limited. And Medicaid coverage, while extensive, is not available to everyone at all times. Also, some facilities provide certain rooms for Medicaid residents and other, better rooms for private paying patients, so that even if Medicaid begins to cover you at some point, you may be forced to move to a different, less desirable room to receive it.

It is very important to find out not only what your coverage is when entering the facility, but also what your personal financial responsibility would be, and how the facility would respond in changing circumstances such as:

- after your allotted Medicare skilled nursing facility coverage is used up;

- moving from skilled to intermediate or personal care, neither of which is covered by Medicare or private insurance;
- becoming eligible for Medicaid if the facility does not accept it;
- personal bankruptcy. Many facilities require proof of your ability to pay for two years as a condition of admission.

Discharge policy: There are situations in which either you anticipate moving out of the facility or the facility wants to discharge you even though you do not necessarily want to leave. Find out the facility's policies and procedures, including how much written notice must be given, in the following and any other discharge situations:

- if the resident's need for care changes and the resident wants to leave the facility to receive different care;
- if the resident's need for care changes and the facility wants the resident to move out and receive care elsewhere, and
- if the resident's source of funds changes.

■

CHECK THE POLICY ON TEMPORARY HOSPITALIZATION

It is not uncommon for a nursing facility resident to require hospitalization for some period of time. Find out what the policy is on holding a resident's bed during hospitalization. If you may be going back and forth to the hospital and you can too easily lose your place in the facility while hospitalized, you may not want that nursing facility.

Now that you have an idea what types of care and facilities are available—and what questions to ask while considering them—you are ready to assess your options for paying for that care.

chapter five

MEDICARE AND VETERANS' BENEFITS

chapter five

MEDICARE AND VETERANS' BENEFITS

Brace yourself for some serious numbers.

Nursing facility care *averaged* $2,500 per month ($30,000 per year) in 1990. Even the less expensive personal care facilities without extensive medical services average over $1,000 per month. And these amounts are increasing much faster than the general cost of living. With such costs, most people exhaust their personal savings within six months of entering a residential care facility. Yet many long-term care residents stay in nursing facilities for two years or more, with total costs reaching more than $100,000. Home health care, too, can run into thousands of dollars a year if services are skilled or frequent.

Who pays for all this? For the most part, the answer is: you pay. And often you pay until your money is gone. A widely-held misconception about the Medicare system is that it "covers" nursing facility care. The truth is that Medicare pays only about two per cent of all nursing facility costs. Medicare coverage for nursing facilities averages less than 30 days of care—and that applies only to skilled nursing care. Medicare covers no long-term nursing facility or other residential care, and its home health care coverage is equally limited.

The idea—increasingly promoted by insurance companies—that private nursing home insurance will protect against the costs of long-term care, is worse than the Medicare myth. It's an outright fraud on the elderly and their families. As discussed in detail in Chapter 10, nursing facility insurance is largely a waste of money and often totally worthless.

The only comprehensive coverage of long-term care comes from Medicaid. This federal government program for low-income people, administered by the states, pays for almost half the nation's total nursing facility costs and for much home care as well. But, as is discussed later (in Chapter 6), a person is not eligible for Medicaid coverage until he or she has used up almost all personal assets. In other words, if you have money saved when you begin long-term care, you must pay the bills yourself until your money is nearly gone; only then will Medicaid begin to pay.

If the alternative of home care is workable for you and your family, little of the cost will be covered by government programs or private insurance. Even so, your out-of-pocket expenses may be lower than for residential care. If you do enter a residential facility, the odds are that you will wind up personally paying for the bulk of care until your assets are nearly gone.

There is no easy way out of this staggering financial crunch. The task is to make your money last as long as possible. You want to be able to use your assets for things other than long-term care. And you want to maintain private assets as long as possible so that you can pay for long-term care services not covered by any government program or insurance.

One way to protect your assets is to buy only the services you really need from the most cost-efficient provider. (See Chapters 1 through 4.) Another approach, discussed in the following chapters, is to take steps to protect your assets before long-term care is necessary, and to get the most coverage from Medicare, Medicaid, other government programs and private insurance if you have it.

The key to getting the most from government programs and insurance coverage is understanding how they work before you commit yourself to a plan of long-term care. The following chapters explain how Medicare and Medicaid programs operate, how private nursing home insurance works—or rather, doesn't work—and what legal and financial steps you can take to protect your assets.

A. MEDICARE COVERAGE FOR LONG-TERM CARE

Most Americans 65 and older are eligible for Medicare coverage, but few understand how it works. Medicare is a federal government program formed to assist older Americans with medical costs. The program is divided into two parts: Part A is "hospital insurance," which covers some bills for a stay in a hospital or a skilled nursing facility; Part B is "medical insurance," which pays some of the costs of doctors and outpatient medical care. If you are 65 or older and eligible for Social Security retirement, survivors or dependents benefits, you are automatically eligible for Part A coverage.[1] And for a monthly premium ($31 in 1989), anyone 65 or older can enroll in Part B coverage, whether or not they are eligible for Part A.

One of the worst misconceptions about Medicare is that it covers nursing facility care. In fact, Medicare nursing facility coverage is severely limited and leaves most people to pay for virtually all long-term care out of their own pockets.

Because home health care can sometimes be considerably cheaper than nursing facility care, it would seem sensible for the government to encourage home care by covering a sizable portion of the cost. Unfortunately, it does not. Medicare pays much less of home care than such logic might lead you to expect, and pays nothing at all for residential care alternatives to nursing homes, such as personal care facilities.

Just as important as knowing what long-term care Medicare does pay for so you can get the most out of available coverage, is knowing what Medicare does *not* pay for so you can be prepared either to gather the funds from somewhere else or to obtain most of your care and coverage from other sources.

1. SKILLED NURSING FACILITY CARE

Part A of Medicare covers a small amount of skilled nursing facility care, as follows:

- up to 100 days per benefit period[2] in a skilled nursing facility;
- a semi-private room (two to four beds); if you want a private room, you must pay for the difference yourself, unless the private room is medically necessary as prescribed by a doctor and approved by the facility and the Medicare intermediary—an

---

[1]Even people who are not eligible for Social Security benefits may be eligible for Part A Medicare when they reach age 65. For a complete discussion of how a person can become eligible for Medicare, see *Social Security, Medicare and Pensions: The Sourcebook for Older Americans* by Joseph Matthews (Nolo Press).

[2]"Benefit period" refers to a continuous period of treatment.

insurance company that administers Medicare funds in your state;[3]

- daily, regular, skilled and special nursing as medically necessary, but *not* a private duty nurse;
- skilled rehabilitation services—such as physical, occupational or speech therapy—as medically necessary and as long as you are showing improvement; and
- medications, medical supplies and equipment, and dietary requirements as supplied by the facility.

■ _____

WARNING—MEDICARE DOES NOT COVER:

- custodial care (non-medical assistance with the normal daily activities such as eating and bathing) unless it is part of skilled nursing care in a skilled nursing facility;
- nursing care or therapy provided in a facility that is not certified by Medicare as a *skilled* nursing facility;[4] or
- doctor's care while you are in a nursing facility. However, Medicare Part B "medical insurance" covers doctor's care in a nursing facility under the same terms as in any other situation.

CONDITIONS LIMITING MEDICARE COVERAGE

Unfortunately, the many conditions placed on Medicare coverage of nursing facility costs eliminate far more care than they cover. When you add these conditions to the fact that Medicare partially pays for a total of only 100 days, it is easy to understand why Medicare pays for only about two per cent of all nursing facility costs.

Immediate prior hospital stay: Medicare pays for a stay in a skilled nursing facility only if you have first spent at least three consecutive days (not counting the discharge day) in a hospital. And

_____

[3]Denial of Medicare coverage can be appealed. The appeal process is described in Medicare pamphlets available from your local Social Security office. There is also a complete explanation of the process in *Social Security, Medicare and Pensions: The Sourcebook for Older Americans* by Joseph Matthews (Nolo Press).

[4]Medicare *may* cover daily skilled nursing care or therapy provided in the skilled nursing section of a multi-level facility if that facility is Medicare-certified and all other conditions are met.

you must be admitted to the nursing facility within 30 days of your discharge from the hospital.

Daily skilled nursing care or therapy: Medicare pays only for the skilled nursing care or rehabilitative therapy you need and receive every day. If you receive such care intermittently, you do not qualify for Medicare coverage because you fail to meet this requirement.

Prescribed by a physician: Your daily skilled nursing care or therapy must be "medically necessary"—specifically prescribed by a doctor.

Medicare-approved skilled nursing facility: You must receive care in a *skilled* nursing facility which is certified by Medicare.[5] And care that is, or could be, received in a lower level facility is not covered.

Only while condition "improving": Even though Medicare could cover up to 100 days in a skilled nursing facility, and even though you may need daily skilled care for all those days, Medicare will cover you only as long as your condition is "improving." Once your condition has stabilized, according to review by Medicare (see below), it will no longer pay for skilled nursing facility care—no matter how serious your condition remains or how much skilled nursing care you continue to need.

Approval on review: The fact that your doctor prescribes "medically necessary" skilled nursing care for you in a skilled nursing facility, and continues to certify that your condition is improving, still does not guarantee that Medicare will provide nursing facility coverage. The doctor's opinion must be approved by both the nursing facility's Utilization Review Committee—facility doctors who review patient conditions—and by the Medicare "intermediary."

HOW MUCH MEDICARE PAYS OF NURSING FACILITY COSTS

During the first 100 days of coverage, Medicare pays the amounts noted below.

---

[5]Medicare checks on the quality of care of each nursing facility and certifies those which meet its standards. Ask to see the current Medicare certification documents of any nursing facility you are considering.

Days 1 to 20: You are responsible for paying up to your yearly Medicare Part A deductible—if you have not already reached it. Once you have paid the yearly deductible, Medicare pays all your covered nursing facility charges.

Days 21-100: After the first 20 days of coverage, Medicare pays all covered charges except what is called a "coinsurance" amount, for which you are personally responsible. For 1989, that coinsurance amount was $25.50 per day; the figure goes up each year.

Days 101 on: After 100 days in a skilled nursing facility you are on your own. Medicare pays nothing toward your stay there.

2. MEDICARE HOME CARE COVERAGE

Although Medicare coverage for home care is extremely limited, it can provide substantial payment for the most expensive part of home care—skilled nursing or therapy—during the time immediately following an illness or injury, when you are most likely to need it.

HOME HEALTH SERVICES COVERED BY MEDICARE

Medicare-covered home health care services are listed below, limited by the conditions discussed in the following section:

- skilled nursing;
- physical and speech therapy: as needed during recovery, while improving;
- supplemental care: if, and only if, you receive skilled nursing or physical or speech therapy, Medicare may also pay for limited visits by a home health care aide to help you with personal care—usually only if there is no one else at home to help. Medicare may also cover required medical social services, some medical supplies or equipment provided by the home care agency, and the services of an occupational therapist to help you relearn daily household tasks.

■
_____

REMINDER

Medicare home health care does *not* cover custodial personal care, drugs, meals or homemaking services.

RESTRICTIONS ON HOME HEALTH CARE COVERAGE

As with nursing facility care, a number of restrictions limit home health care coverage. Medicare applies only during periods of recovery from acute illness or injury, or following a change in condition while you are learning how to administer drugs or otherwise care for yourself. Intermittent skilled care: It must be "medically necessary" for you to receive skilled nursing care or rehabilitative therapy on a *part-time only* basis. Full-time nursing care at home is not covered. Note that this is the opposite of the requirement for such care in a skilled nursing facility.

Doctor-prescribed: The skilled care must have been ordered by a physician.

Only during recovery: Care is covered only while you are recovering—that is, while your condition is improving. As soon as your condition has stabilized, as determined by a Medicare review, coverage ends.

Injury, illness or medical condition: Your need for care must be the result of a specific injury, illness or medical condition. If it is the result of general frailness, Medicare will not cover home care.

Confined to home: Care is covered only while you are confined to home except for brief, infrequent occasions out, usually related to receiving medical care. "Confined to home" is defined as being unable to leave home without difficulty and without the assistance of another person or a medical device such as a wheelchair. Confined to home does *not* necessarily mean bedridden, however.

Approved agency: Care must be provided by a Medicare-certified home care agency or other provider. This sometimes eliminates independent nurses and therapists. Always ask the home care agency or other provider to show you its Medicare certification documentation *before* beginning care.

HOW MUCH MEDICARE HOME HEALTH COVERAGE PAYS

In general, Medicare pays 100% of the "approved costs" of the *covered* services provided by a certified home care agency or other provider. "Approved costs" are the standardized charges Medicare decides are appropriate for specific services, based on a national cost average. You are personally responsible for the cost of any non-covered services such as homemaking or unapproved personal care from a home care aide.

No matter what the home care provider might normally charge for the covered services, it must accept as payment in full whatever Medicare decides is the approved cost. The home care agency will submit all bills for covered services directly to Medicare. You don't have to be involved in the paperwork.

In some situations, it may not be clear whether Medicare will cover a particular service. In that case, the home care agency or other provider must notify you in writing of that doubt *before* it provides the service. If it does notify you and you accept the service anyway but Medicare denies coverage, you are personally responsible for the bill. If it does *not* notify you in advance, the provider cannot bill you.

■ —————————————————————————————————————

MEDI-GAP PRIVATE SUPPLEMENTAL INSURANCE

Many people have private health insurance policies designed to supplement Medicare coverage, commonly called "Medi-gap" policies. A few of these policies have provisions for skilled nursing facility or home health care coverage. But almost all of them cover no more of nursing facility or home health care services than Medicare does. If Medicare doesn't cover a service, you can be pretty sure the Medi-gap policy doesn't cover it either. If it is covered, the Medi-gap policy will pay only the percentage of approved Medicare costs Medicare does not pay. In most cases, then, the Medi-gap policy will pay very little, but of course it can be helpful.

Check your Medi-gap policy to see if it provides any nursing facility or home health care coverage. Even if coverage seems unlikely, it doesn't hurt to file a claim and see what coverage you can get. After all, you've paid for it. (See Chapter 10 for a detailed discussion of Medi-gap insurance.)

B. VETERANS' BENEFITS FOR LONG-TERM CARE

The Veterans' Administration operates more than 150 hospitals and a number of outpatient clinics throughout the United States that provide free or very low-cost health care for veterans and their dependents. The care at these facilities is usually very good, but in-patient care is limited. Although there are many hospitals and over 100,000 beds, there are millions of veterans and their dependents, so the VA reserves in-patient care for the treatment of acute conditions, with priority to service-connected illness and injury and to veterans who cannot afford care elsewhere. Some space for in-patient long-term care for the elderly is available, but it is severely limited.

1. ELIGIBILITY FOR VETERANS' BENEFITS

Many elders may be eligible for Veterans' Administration medical benefits based on their military service or their spouse's service even if their current need for long-term care has nothing to do with any service-connected disability.[6]

In general, any veteran is eligible for medical care from a VA facility if unable to afford care elsewhere. Dependents and survivors of veterans with service-connected disabilities, or those who receive veterans' pensions or are eligible for Medicaid, are also eligible to receive medical care from VA facilities if they are unable to afford the care elsewhere.

2. HOME HEALTH CARE COVERED BY VETERANS' BENEFITS

There are more and more home health care units connected to Veterans' Administration hospitals and clinics. And the care is free of

---

[6]Disability compensation for "service-connected disability" and pension benefits for financially needy veterans are not discussed here, but may be available as extra sources of income. Check with your local Veterans' Administration for eligibility.

charge. But unless there is such a home care unit in your area, the VA will rarely pay for care provided by an outside agency.[7]

If a VA facility near you has a home health care unit, it can provide complete medical and personal care as often as necessary. The period of care is usually limited to recovery from acute illness, injury or surgery, but if specific medical care is needed, it may be available on a long-term basis.

So, if you are a veteran or dependent or survivor of a veteran who needs home health care, contact your local VA office to find out if home care is available from a facility in your area. If it is, it may well be worth finding out about eligibility and coverage.

3. NURSING FACILITY CARE COVERED BY VETERANS' BENEFITS

A number of VA facilities provide long-term skilled nursing and intermediate residential care for veterans. In general, simple custodial care without the need for regular nursing or other health care is not available, but where the VA draws the line in a given case may depend on the availability of beds in a particular facility.

VA coverage for skilled or intermediate care in a private facility is sometimes possible if similar care is not available in a VA facility. Eligibility depends on financial need as well as any connection between the disability or impairment and military service. Because the quality of free VA health care tends to be very good while costing the veteran nothing, it is worth it to investigate both your eligibility and the availability of long-term residential care in a VA facility. The search for information should begin with your local VA office and with any VA medical facility in your area.

---

[7]If you have a 50% or higher rated service-connected disability, the VA *may* cover some home health care from a non-VA agency. But you must obtain prior approval from the VA.

MEDICAID COVERAGE FOR LONG-TERM CARE

MEDICAID COVERAGE FOR LONG-TERM CARE

Medicaid[1] is a federally-funded program, administered by the individual states, which helps pay for medical care for financially needy people. For low-income older people who qualify, Medicaid supplements Medicare to cover many long-term costs Medicare does not—including home care and almost all levels of nursing facility care for an unlimited time. The Medicaid program pays for about half of the country's total nursing facility costs.

To qualify for Medicaid, an elder must have a low income and very few assets. Unfortunately, this means that many people are not eligible until they have used up almost all their savings paying for nursing facility or home care themselves.

Another problem with Medicaid nursing facility coverage is that many facilities either do not accept Medicaid residents, or put them only in less desirable rooms, because Medicaid pays a lower rate than that charged to privately-paying residents. So, if you are dependent on Medicaid when you enter a nursing facility, your choices may be limited. And if your funds diminish to the point that you become eligible for Medicaid after you are a resident, although by law the facility cannot discharge you, it might move you to a different room. Before choosing a nursing facility, find out the details of its Medicaid policy.

---

[1]Called Medi-Cal in California.

A NOTE ON FINANCIAL PLANNING

As discussed below, Medicaid eligibility rules severely restrict how much people can keep of their lifetime savings. Chapter 7 discusses ways you may be able to protect some of your assets and still qualify for Medicaid. Even if you are not yet eligible for Medicaid or not yet considering residence in a nursing facility, read both this chapter and the next one carefully. Planning could save you many thousands of dollars in the future, and allow you to do what you would like with the money instead of handing it over to a nursing facility.

A. ELIGIBILITY FOR MEDICAID

Each state has its own Medicaid eligibility standards, so check with your county's social services agency for the rules in your state. Overall federal government standards require your assets and income to be below certain levels, with special rules for nursing facility residents, which differ greatly for unmarried[2] individuals and married couples.

1. HOME CARE INCOME AND ASSET LIMITS

The following are the general federal guidelines for the amount of income and assets—savings, investment, property—a person receiving care who is not a resident of a nursing facility is allowed to keep and still receive Medicaid funds. Some states have stricter rules, other states are more liberal. If you are close to these figures, be sure to apply.

INCOME LIMITS

An individual can have a monthly income of around $300 to $500 and still qualify for Medicaid; for a couple, the figure is roughly $500 to $700. Income includes Social Security and other government benefits, wages or self-employment income, interest or dividends from savings

---

[2]"Unmarried" does not necessarily mean never married; it also refers to people who are divorced or have no spouse living.

and investments, rents, royalties, pensions, annuities and gifts. If one spouse is still working, though, the first $65 per month of earned income (wages or self-employment) plus one-half of all amounts over that is not counted toward these income limits.

ASSET LIMITS

People who are not residents of a nursing facility may have non-exempt assets of no more than $2,000 ($3,000 for a couple). Fortunately, a number of assets are exempted from these figures. The most significant exempt asset is your home, if either you or your spouse live in it. Also exempted are your car up to a value of $4,500 and up to $2,000 worth of household goods and personal effects. Again, these are approximate figures and you must check with your local county social services office to find out the specific rules in your state.

WHOSE MONEY COUNTS?

Medicaid has a number of rules for counting assets and income to determine eligibility:

- The assets and income of children, grandchildren or other relatives do not count toward Medicaid limits, even if they live in the same household as the elder applying for Medicaid, except to the extent they provide regular financial support. Regular financial support is not limited to money but can include food and clothing or other personal items.
- If a married couple live together, both of their incomes and assets are counted toward the Medicaid limits.
- If a couple is divorced or legally separated and living apart, then only the income and assets of the spouse applying for Medicaid are counted, including any actual support received from the other spouse.
- If a couple live together but are not married, only the income and assets of the person applying for Medicaid are counted, including any direct financial support received from the other partner.

■ ──

DISPOSING OF ASSETS

People often try to preserve some of their assets while keeping their eligibility for Medicaid. They give assets to children or other relatives or friends before applying to Medicaid. And some married couples go so far as to get divorced, particularly if they will be entering a nursing facility, since the cost of being a private resident can quickly eat up even large savings.

Medicaid regulations make it difficult to save assets, and people who do not know the rules in advance almost always make mistakes that cost them their assets or eligibility. But there are several legal ways to preserve some assets and still qualify for Medicaid coverage. These methods are discussed in detail in Chapter 7.

2. SPECIAL NURSING FACILITY MEDICAID RULES

Once a nursing facility resident has qualified, Medicaid pays virtually all facility costs for as long as a person remains there. But as with home care, a nursing facility resident is only eligible when his or her assets are below a certain level. Until then, the resident must pay. Once Medicaid begins paying, almost all of an individual's or a couple's income will go to the nursing home to reduce the amounts Medicaid pays.

Because Medicaid rules for nursing facility residents are quite different for unmarried individuals and for couples, this section is divided in two parts. The first section explains the income and assets which can be retained by a single person who enters a nursing facility. The second section explains the income and assets that each member of a married couple can retain when one spouse enters a nursing facility.

UNMARRIED INDIVIDUALS IN A NURSING FACILITY

Remember that for Medicaid purposes, "unmarried" includes those who are divorced or whose spouse has died. Also, beware that if your marital status changes after you qualify for Medicaid, the Medicaid limits on your income and assets will also change.

INCOME ELIGIBILITY LIMITS

About 30 states have no limits at all on the income a nursing facility resident can have and still be eligible for Medicaid coverage. But note that, as discussed below, virtually all of that income will go to the nursing facility, with Medicaid paying the balance of the cost.

The rest of the states do have eligibility income limits, which vary from about $700 to $1,100 per month. A nursing facility resident in one of these states with an income over the limit does not qualify for Medicaid coverage at all.

■ _____

STATES WITH INCOME TEST FOR MEDICAID ELIGIBILITY

Alabama	Nevada
Alaska	New Jersey
Arkansas	New Mexico
Colorado	Oklahoma
Delaware	South Carolina
Florida	South Dakota
Georgia	Tennessee
Idaho	Texas
Iowa	Wyoming
Louisiana	

INCOME RETAINED BY THE RESIDENT

If an unmarried nursing facility resident qualifies for Medicaid, all of that person's monthly income will go to the nursing facility, with Medicaid paying the balance of the nursing facility bill, except:

- A small monthly amount for personal needs—books and magazines, grooming and toilet articles—with the total value ranging from $30 to $70, depending on the state.
- Credit is given toward the nursing facility bill for income the resident spends directly on Medicare premiums, deductibles and co-payments, on medical insurance and on out-of-pocket medical expenses not covered by Medicare or Medicaid.
- In about 30 states, a resident can keep $150 to $600 a month for upkeep and repairs on his or her private residence. This home

maintenance allowance is permitted for up to six months upon a written prognosis by the resident's doctor that the resident is expected to be able to return home from the nursing facility within six months after entering it.

ASSET ELIGIBILITY LIMITS

Before Medicaid will cover an unmarried person's stay in a nursing facility, that person's savings and other assets must be reduced to certain limits. If your assets exceed these limits, you will qualify for Medicaid coverage only after you have paid for nursing facility coverage out of your own pocket—referred to by Medicaid as "spending down"—until you reach these limits.[3] The Medicaid limits allow:

- no more than $2,000 in savings or other liquid assets such as stocks or certificates of deposit. This limit varies slightly from state to state;
- household and personal items up to a value of about $2,000;
- one automobile up to a value of $4,500;
- one wedding and one engagement ring of any value;
- a burial plot and up to $1,500 in a separately maintained fund for burial costs;
- a life insurance policy with a face value of no more than $1,500;
- a home, under limited circumstances. In most states, a home will not be counted in determining Medicaid eligibility for nursing facility coverage only if your doctor certifies in writing that you are likely to recover sufficiently to leave the nursing facility and return home. Some states also add a six- to twelve-month time limit, no matter what your doctor says.

---

[3]Medicaid rules do not permit you to simply "give away" assets to relatives or friends and then qualify for coverage. Ways to protect your assets and still qualify for Medicaid, however, are discussed in detail in Chapter 7.

■
_____

HOW DOES MEDICAID KNOW WHAT YOUR ASSETS ARE?

A natural question arises when people read that Medicaid coverage is available only to people whose assets are below certain levels: How does Medicaid know what my assets are?

The answer is that when you apply for Medicaid, you fill out extensive application forms that ask you to list all your assets. You must also show the Medicaid eligibility workers copies of all ownership documents, bank books and the like. If there are any large withdrawals from your assets in the 30 months prior to your application, you will have to prove where that money went and why. Remember, too, that Medicaid will have your Social Security number, so it can cross-check many financial transactions. Medicaid eligibility workers can also pay home visits.

If you fail to report income or assets and are caught by Medicaid, you run the risk of being denied coverage, being forced to repay any money already paid on your behalf and even facing criminal and civil penalties.

MARRIED COUPLES WITH ONE SPOUSE IN A NURSING FACILITY

While most states do not set income limits for unmarried people entering a nursing facility, there are different rules for couples. Many states set limits for couples when one spouse is in a nursing facility.

WHOSE INCOME COUNTS FOR ELIGIBILITY?

Most states use a "name-on-the-check" rule to determine whether income received by a married couple is counted against the Medicaid eligibility of the spouse in the nursing facility. This rule basically says that if the income is received in the name of the at-home spouse, it is not counted toward the state's maximum income limit for the nursing facility spouse's Medicaid eligibility.

Two states—California and Washington—have "community property" rules, which can help a nursing facility spouse qualify for Medicaid coverage when the name-on-the-check rule would deny eligibility. If the nursing facility spouse in a community property state receives income in his or her name that is over the state's Medicaid limit, Medicaid will see how much income is received in the name of the at-home spouse as well. If one-half the total community property income (the combined income received in the name of both spouses) is not over the limit, then the nursing facility spouse will qualify for Medicaid even though the name-on-the-check rule would have denied eligibility.

Three other states—Indiana, Nebraska and West Virginia—also count the at-home spouse's income over certain limits as part of the nursing facility spouse's income when calculating eligibility.

INCOME RETAINED BY EACH SPOUSE

Of income received in his or her own name, the nursing facility spouse may keep between $30 to $70 per month for personal use, plus amounts to pay for Medicare, other medical insurance and medical expenses not covered by Medicare or Medicaid. The rest of the income in the name of the nursing facility spouse goes to the nursing facility, except for an amount needed to meet the at-home spouse's minimum allowance. The at-home spouse is allowed to keep all income in his or her own name. If more than half the couple's joint income is in the nursing facility spouse's name, the at-home spouse is allowed to keep some of the income in the nursing facility spouse's name up to a basic living allowance of between $750 and $1,500 per month, combining the two incomes. The specific amount varies from state to state. Check with the local social services agency to find out the limits in your state.

ASSETS RETAINED BY BOTH SPOUSES

The name-on-the-check rule does not apply to assets—savings, property, investments. It used to be true that if a couple transferred all their assets to the sole name of the at-home spouse, the nursing facility spouse might qualify for Medicaid. No longer. Medicaid now looks at the combined assets of both spouses, although some property transfers may still be possible. Although the amounts vary a bit from state to state, in general the combined assets a couple may retain and still qualify for Medicaid coverage of the nursing facility spouse are:

- the home in which the at-home spouse lives, regardless of its value.

- one automobile, regardless of its value;
- furniture and household goods, regardless of value;
- one wedding and engagement ring each, regardless of value;
- life insurance with face value (the amount it would bring if cashed in) of $1,500;
- two burial plots and a separate savings account of up to $1,500 for each person for burial costs;
- up to $6,000 of property (such as tools or equipment) required for the support of the at-home spouse; and
- one-half the value of all other assets at the time the nursing facility spouse enters the nursing facility. Each state sets its own limit, from a low of $12,000 up to a maximum of $60,000.

Note: It is important to establish the total value of your assets through bank records or other documentation when the nursing facility spouse enters a nursing facility so that you can claim and retain one-half the full value.

REMINDER ABOUT TRANSFERS OF PROPERTY

Most transfers of property made to get under eligibility limits are not valid under Medicaid rules, but there are a few legal ways to protect assets. Some of the most effective methods must be started before a spouse enters a nursing facility. See Chapter 7 for a complete discussion of how to protect your savings and other assets.

B. WHAT MEDICAID PAYS FOR

As with eligibility, what Medicaid covers and how much it pays varies by state. In general, though, Medicaid pays for broader home care coverage than Medicare and much more of nursing facility care.

1. MEDICAID-CERTIFIED PROVIDERS ONLY

Medicaid pays only for covered services performed by a Medicaid-certified provider. Some agencies and facilities do not meet Medicaid quality standards and therefore are not certified to participate in the program. Also, because Medicaid pays less than what agencies or facilities charge private consumers, some providers choose not to participate in the Medicaid program.[4] And some home care providers either do not meet Medicaid standards or choose not to participate because of Medicaid paperwork or wanting to be paid in cash.

It is important to find out whether a provider participates in Medicaid before you obtain service from it. This is particularly true for nursing facility residence. Even if you are not initially dependent on Medicaid, find out the facility's policy on Medicaid patients. Some facilities maintain different, less desirable rooms for Medicaid patients. Switching to Medicaid later may affect the quality of care you receive.

2. MEDICAID HOME CARE COVERAGE

Unlike Medicare, Medicaid does not usually have stringent rules about either the kind or duration of home care services it covers. In most states, Medicaid pays most of a certified home care agency's reasonable costs, even if care is primarily custodial, and covers many services by non-agency providers, as long as they are Medicaid-certified. In some states, Medicaid also pays for extra-duty nursing, rehabilitation therapies provided outside the home, prescribed medications and medical supplies. To find out whether Medicaid covers a particular service in your state, check with both the provider of the service and your local social service office.

If Medicaid covers a service and the provider accepts payment from Medicaid, the provider cannot then charge you for any amounts over that payment. But, of course, the provider can and will charge you for services not covered by Medicaid.

In some states, Medicaid charges additional fees as noted below.

---

[4]Some facilities will accept only private paying residents but will permit a resident to remain after he or she has switched to Medicaid coverage.

- **Enrollment Fee:** Some states charge a small, one-time only fee of a few dollars when you first enroll in Medicaid.
- **Monthly Premium:** States are allowed to charge a small fee to "medically needy" Medicaid participants—those who would not normally qualify because of their income or assets, but who become eligible because paying their medical bills would drop their income or assets below the eligibility levels. The amounts of these premiums vary but are usually only two or three dollars a month.
- **Co-payments:** States may charge a co-payment—as Medicare does for the first few days of nursing facility care—which is a fixed amount for each covered service you receive. This may be charged only to those who qualify for Medicaid as "medically needy" (see above) or to any Medicaid recipient of services the state Medicaid program is not required by federal law to cover, but which it covers anyway as an "optional" service.

3. MEDICAID NURSING FACILITY COVERAGE

Unlike Medicare, Medicaid can be a lifesaver when it comes to nursing facility bills. In general, Medicaid pays for all levels of care in certified facilities for an indefinite period of time.

LEVELS OF CARE COVERED

Medicaid in all states covers residence in certified skilled nursing facilities. But unlike Medicare, coverage does not require a prior hospital stay.

The greatest advantage Medicaid has over Medicare coverage is that many state Medicaid programs also cover residence in certified intermediate care and personal care facilities. This means that Medicaid coverage exists for the situation that most commonly exhausts a family's savings: a long-term stay in a personal care facility where the resident receives primarily non-medical custodial care.

Unlike Medicare, Medicaid coverage is not limited to a certain number of days. Medicaid covers nursing facility residence indefinitely, although it will frequently review the level of care being received and may require that residence be shifted to a lower-level care facility if it determines a higher level of care is no longer medically necessary.

HOW MUCH MEDICAID PAYS

Some state Medicaid programs pay only a certain percentage of the cost of care. Check in advance with both the facility and your local Medicaid social worker to determine what Medicaid will cover and how much it will pay.

In general, Medicaid pays a nursing or other qualifying residential facility a daily rate that covers medical and personal or custodial care, rehabilitation therapies provided by the facility, and room and board. And for whatever Medicaid covers, the facility must accept Medicaid's payment as payment in full. The facility cannot bill you for any additional amounts for covered services. However, the facility can bill you personally for services not covered by Medicaid in your state, such as personal supplies, some medicines and non-covered services from outside providers, such as clothes cleaning, hair dressing or a visit from a dental hygienist.

C. FINDING OUT ABOUT MEDICAID IN YOUR STATE

■
_____

REMINDER

Before you apply for Medicaid, read Chapter 7 and take the steps explained there that could help protect your assets from nursing facility and other costs.

To qualify for Medicaid, you must file a written application to the agency that handles Medicaid on the local level, usually the county Department of Social Services, Health Department or Welfare Department. If you or a family member are already hospitalized or in a nursing facility, ask to have the medical social worker assist you in obtaining and filling out the applications.

There are a number of documents you should bring with you when you apply, most of which have to do with your financial situation. Even if you do not have the following documents, go ahead and begin the application process. The Medicaid eligibility workers can help you get whatever papers and documents are necessary, including:

- most recent interest and dividend statements, previous year's income tax return, recent pension and Social Security benefit papers or deposit slips indicating your current income;
- papers showing all your financial assets, such as bank books, insurance policies, stock certificates and car registration. If you used the assets worksheet in Chapter 1, bring documents reflecting all the assets you listed there;
- rent receipts, lease agreement or canceled rent checks if you are a renter, or mortgage payment book and latest tax assessment on the property if you're a home owner;
- your Social Security card or number;
- if you live with your spouse, information about his or her income and separate assets; and
- medical bills from the previous three months. And if you are planning on home care or residence in a care facility in the near future, bring medical records or reports that confirm your condition will require the particular care. If you don't have records or reports, bring the names and addresses of doctors who are treating you.

You will be interviewed and assisted in filling out your application by a Medicaid eligibility worker. Write down his or her name and telephone extension in case you have specific questions during the application process.

It may take several visits and there may be delays in processing your application while the proper documents are located and reviewed. Normally you will receive a decision within a few weeks; the law says a decision must be made within 45 days after your application is complete. If you don't hear from Medicaid within 30 days after completing your application, call the Medicaid social worker who interviewed you and ask what's going on. Social service and Medicaid agencies are very overworked and sometimes a person's application gets delayed in the shuffle. Stay on top of things so your application isn't delayed any more than necessary.

■
_____

THE RETROACTIVE COVERAGE RULE

A valuable rule says that if you become eligible for Medicaid, you may be covered for home care or nursing facility costs back to the beginning of the third month before you filed your application. You must present proof of covered costs during that time. Make sure when you apply that your Medicaid eligibility worker knows you want retroactive coverage.

D. WHAT TO DO IF YOU ARE DENIED MEDICAID COVERAGE

If you are notified that you do not qualify for Medicaid, or that coverage is denied for a particular service, facility or time period, you have a right to what is called a "fair hearing" to determine if the decision is correct. If you receive notice of a decision you do not agree with, inquire immediately, at the office where you applied, about the procedure in your state for getting a fair hearing.

The rules for a fair hearing vary, but in general you are permitted to have a friend, relative, social worker, lawyer or other representative appear with you and testify about your financial situation, medical condition or expenses if such evidence would be helpful. The hearing itself is informal and you will be able to explain your position in your own words, without having to worry about legal technicalities or jargon. If your medical condition or need for treatment is the crucial question, a detailed letter from your doctor would be of great help. The hearing officer who makes the decision is not a judge but is a Medicaid eligibility specialist.

Although the odds of getting a Medicaid denial reversed at a fair hearing are not in your favor, such reversals do happen frequently enough, and the amount of money involved is large enough, that it is worth the effort. And even if the fair hearing officer decides against you, there may be procedures in your state for further appeal. Information about that appeal will probably be given to you along with the fair hearing decision. If not, check with your local social service office.

■

FREE ASSISTANCE GETTING NURSING FACILITY COVERAGE

If you are entering a nursing or personal care facility and are having trouble either being accepted for Medicaid or getting Medicaid to cover that facility, contact your state's Nursing Home Ombudsman. The ombudsman program is financed by the federal government and its purpose is to assist people with problems relating to nursing facilities. There is no charge for using its services. You can find your local office of the Nursing Home Ombudsman under that name in the white pages of your telephone directory, or through the Senior Information and Referral. You can also be referred to the ombudsman through your area, state or local Agency on Aging, or through the central ombudsman office for your state. (See the Resource Directory in the Appendix at the back of this book.)

PROTECTING YOUR ASSETS

PROTECTING YOUR ASSETS

A. MEDICAID RULES ON TRANSFER OF ASSETS

As discussed in Chapter 6, a person is only eligible for Medicaid when his or her assets are reduced to minimum levels, which vary from state to state and also with marital status. A person (and spouse) must personally pay home care, nursing facility or other costs until assets are reduced to Medicaid levels. In many cases, this means that entering a nursing facility wipes out most of a life's savings before Medicaid begins paying at all.

To avoid spending all their savings on nursing facility care before Medicaid begins coverage, many people used to give away assets—or at least transfer legal title—to children or other relatives, then apply for Medicaid. But Medicaid rules now severely restrict such transfers. Today, it takes careful planning to avoid having most of your assets eaten up by the costs of long-term care. And some protective transfers are only possible if you are willing to give control of the assets to your children or others and trust them to manage the assets for you.

But before learning about some ways to avoid the harsh consequences of Medicaid rules, it is important to understand what property transfers those rules permit.

1. FORBIDDEN TRANSFERS

There is one basic Medicaid rule limiting the transfer of assets by nursing facility residents: Anything transferred from your name during the 30 months before either applying for Medicaid, or entering a nursing facility if you are already receiving Medicaid, is considered an invalid transfer. The effect of this invalid transfer rule is that your eligibility for Medicaid is delayed for a period of time (no longer than

30 months) determined by the value of the asset transferred, divided by the average monthly nursing facility cost in your state.

Example: You transfer a certificate of deposit worth $10,000 to your daughter within the 30 month-period before you apply for Medicaid. If the average monthly nursing facility cost in your state is $2,000, the $10,000 you transferred would be divided by the $2,000 monthly average cost, meaning you would be ineligible for Medicaid for a period of five months (10,000 divided by 2,000 = 5).

2. PERMISSIBLE TRANSFERS

Medicaid permits some exceptions to this 30-month rule. These can be of particular benefit to a married couple with one spouse entering a nursing facility. Read these rules *carefully*. A little planning may save you a lot of money.

As soon as you, a spouse or other relative begin to consider the possibility of entering a nursing facility, it is time to plan transfers of assets. (See Section B, Protecting Assets from Nursing Facility Costs, for help.)

UNMARRIED INDIVIDUALS

Either *before or after entering a nursing facility*, an unmarried person can transfer the assets listed below without any eligibility penalty.

Home. A home can be transferred:

- to a minor child (through a custodianship or trust arrangement), or to a blind or disabled child of any age;
- to a child of any age who has lived in the home for two years prior to the parent's entry into a nursing facility and who cared for the parent, allowing the parent to remain at home rather than enter a nursing facility during that time;
- to a brother or sister who already has some ownership interest in the property and who has lived in the home for at least the previous year.

Exempt assets. You may transfer to anyone, at any time, your car worth up to $4,500, personal or household belongings worth up to $2,000, your engagement or wedding rings, or other exempt assets. (See the list of exempt assets in Chapter 6.)

Non-exempt assets. You may transfer any asset, at any time, to a minor, blind or disabled child. You may also transfer any asset at any time to any person if you can prove to Medicaid that the purpose of the transfer was something *other* than to qualify for Medicaid, such as to help a relative in need.

MARRIED PEOPLE ENTERING A NURSING FACILITY

Medicaid rules give married couples two advantages over unmarried people in protecting assets: one permits protecting a home; the other permits protecting *any* asset if the timing of the transfer is just right.

Home. A married person can transfer title to a home to his or her spouse either before or after entering a nursing facility. Although the home is exempt anyway as long as the spouse is living in it, as is discussed more fully later in this chapter, it may be best to transfer title to the at-home spouse, who can then transfer the home to children or others in case the at-home spouse should die first. A married person can also transfer title to the home to any of the other people an unmarried person can transfer to, as described above.

Exempt Assets. A married person at any time can transfer exempt assets to anyone. (Refer to Chapter 6 for the list of a married couple's exempt assets.)

Other Assets. Any assets, at any time, can be transferred to a minor, blind or disabled child. Any asset can also be transferred to anyone at any time if it can be *proved* by the person transferring that the transfer was for some purpose other than to qualify for Medicaid. Such proof is difficult, however, and would require convincing testimony as to the validity of the reason for the transfer—for example, to help a brother or sister keep a failing business, or to pay a child's uninsured medical costs.

Before entering a nursing facility, a spouse may transfer any asset to his or her at-home spouse, but *only if* the at-home spouse does not transfer it to anyone else within 30 months, for less than its true value. For example, title to assets cannot be transferred to the sole name of the at-home spouse and then given immediately to the children.

After entering a nursing facility, but *before* applying for Medicaid, you can take advantage of a loophole in the Medicaid rules that permits the nursing facility spouse to transfer any asset to the other spouse, who can then transfer it to anyone else without Medicaid penalty if all transfers are completed before applying for Medicaid.

■

IMPORTANT

This last rule may be extremely useful if a couple has children or other people they trust to manage their assets for them. With a little planning, they can save their assets no matter how large— although it means giving up control over them—and still get Medicaid coverage without waiting 30 months. Preparations for transferring title to the at-home spouse should be made before entering the nursing facility. But one spouse must actually become a nursing facility resident before, in the following order:
1. transferring the assets to the at-home spouse;
2. the assets are transferred out of the at-home spouse's name; and
3. applying for Medicaid.
(See below for a complete discussion of this procedure.)

B. PROTECTING ASSETS FROM NURSING FACILITY COSTS

Although Medicaid rules require you to use up most of your assets paying for nursing facility care before Medicaid begins to pay, there are ways to preserve many of those assets. Each option has some drawbacks, however, and not all of them will be available for everyone. Different methods pertain to unmarried people and to couples; some require advanced planning and perhaps the assistance of a lawyer or other professional adviser. Read carefully through all these suggestions before you decide which might be right for you.

1. INVESTMENTS IN YOUR HOME

Because Medicaid rules often exempt a home of any value from asset eligibility limits, concentrating your assets in your home is a good way to protect them. This is useful for both unmarried individuals and for couples, but the rules are different for each and must be carefully followed. Assuming you don't have other immediate needs for your savings or investments, you could put those assets into your home by:

- paying off your outstanding mortgage;
- making home improvements or building additions; or by
- buying a new home or condominium for more money than your present home is worth. For the home to be protected, though, you or your spouse must live in it.

HOME INVESTMENT BY INDIVIDUALS

The ways in which an unmarried individual can protect assets through his or her home are very limited and may require some professional assistance from a lawyer or tax accountant.

States with no return home rule. Medicaid rules in a few states permit unmarried nursing facility residents to exempt their homes without requiring a doctor's certification that their physical condition is likely to improve to the extent that they can return home to live. If you live in a state with no "return home rule," you may be free to protect assets by investing them in your home, as described above.

Exempt child or sibling. If your adult child or brother or sister lives in your home and would qualify the home as an exempt asset, you may want to invest further in the home. (See the explanation, above.)

Transfer to non-exempt adult child. Even if it would not qualify the house as an exempt asset, you may still want to consider investing assets in the house and transferring title to a son or daughter. This means giving up control over the property, so you must trust your child to manage it according to your wishes. Also, you must want the home to remain that child's property after your death.

The benefit of transferring your home to your child comes from not having to sell the home to pay your own nursing facility bills. If you transfer the home more than 30 months before you apply for Medicaid or enter a nursing facility, the value of the home will not affect your Medicaid eligibility at all. If you transfer it within 30 months of entering a nursing facility, your eligibility will be delayed for a period equal to the value of the home divided by the average monthly nursing facility in your state, up to a maximum of 30 months. (See the explanation of the Medicaid 30-month rule in Section A1 of this chapter.) Unless you have equity in your home of less than about $60,000, such a transfer would almost always result in a delay in Medicaid coverage for the full 30 months.

Creating a life estate. A "life estate" is a legal maneuver that transfers title to property, without affecting who has use of the property.

Here's how it works. A legal document is drawn up creating a life estate in the home, which permits the elder to live there for the rest of his or her life.[1] The life estate "remainder"—the value remaining after the death of the homeowner—goes to the homeowner's children, or any other person designated, upon the homeowner's death.

The Medicaid advantage of a life estate is that in calculating an unmarried person's assets, most states normally count the full value of the home. The homeowner must sell it and use the funds to pay for nursing facility care before becoming eligible for Medicaid. With a life estate, the elder no longer has the value of the home as an asset, but only has the value of remaining there for life. If a person must enter a nursing facility with the possibility of not returning home, and if returning, of not living many years there, then the value of the life estate is far smaller than the value of the home. The elder would only be required to spend an amount equal to the value of the life estate, rather than the greater value of the home, before being eligible for Medicaid.

---

[1]You will probably need the help of a lawyer to ensure that a life estate is created properly. Also, advice may be needed on the possible tax consequences for the person to whom the property is transferred.

■

TAX CONSEQUENCES OF PROPERTY TRANSFERS

Transferring your home or other valuable assets may have
unforeseen gift tax and income tax consequences. In general, an
individual can make a gift valued up to $10,000 to another
individual each year without any gift tax consequences. For
example, if there are six people to whom you wish to make gifts
(four adult children and two spouses of those children) you
could make gifts totaling $60,000 per year. In addition, there is
no gift tax for any amounts left to someone at death but given
away to that person during one's lifetime if the total estate at
death is valued under $600,000.

Income tax consequences have to do with the tax basis of
the property, which is usually lower if property is given away
upon death.

See Chapter 9 for a more detailed discussion of tax basis
rules.

HOME INVESTMENT BY COUPLES

A home is a particularly good place for a married couple to invest
savings or other assets. Even if one spouse enters a nursing facility, as
long as the other spouse lives at home, it is completely exempt from
Medicaid eligibility limits no matter how much it is worth.

Investing in the home may only be the beginning of protecting
assets there. But additional steps can be taken to further protect those
assets:

Title transfer to spouse. If one spouse enters a nursing
facility, he or she should transfer sole title to the property to the spouse
who remains at home. The spouse at home should then create a "living
trust" that leaves the home to children or anyone else other than the
nursing facility spouse. (See Chapter 9 for a more detailed discussion of
living trusts.) If the at-home spouse dies first, or moves out of the
home, under the terms of the living trust, the home would go to the
beneficiaries of the trust. If title to the home is left jointly in the name
of the nursing facility spouse, when the at-home spouse dies or enters
a nursing facility, Medicaid rules require the value of the home to go to
the nursing facility and not to the children or other beneficiaries.

Also, once the home is in the sole name of the at-home spouse, he or she may be able to make good use of its equity, for example, by selling the home and using the money. There are also other equity conversion devices, such as reverse annuity mortgages in which a home with a large amount of equity is used as collateral for a loan and the lender makes monthly or lump sum payments to the homeowner. One such method might provide income, some of which could be protected from Medicaid consideration.

To know what transfer of title, sale of your home, living trusts or equity conversion devices might mean for you in terms of tax advantages and disadvantages measured against Medicaid eligibility, it is recommended that you seek the advice of a lawyer, accountant, or business adviser who is familiar with both Medicaid rules and tax laws.

■

DURABLE POWERS OF ATTORNEY: PROTECTION FOR TRANSFERABILITY

A number of the methods for protecting assets require that a spouse in a nursing facility make legal transfers of property. Such transfers are only possible, however, if the spouse still has legal capacity—which basically means soundness of mind or mental competence. A stroke or other sudden onset of disease can eliminate that legal capacity without warning. It is usually wise for all older people with assets to consider having "durable powers of attorney," which permit others to make legal decisions if and when someone becomes incapacitated. (Durable powers of attorney are discussed fully in Chapter 8.)

2. INVESTING IN OTHER EXEMPT ASSETS

A home is not the only asset automatically exempt from Medicaid eligibility limits. Those listed below are also exempt, and up to each state's limits, can be invested in without being touched by the nursing facility:

- an automobile (up to $4,500 for an individual, of any value for a couple);

■ furniture and household goods (up to $2,000 for an individual, of any value for a couple);

■ one wedding and one engagement ring per person of any value (individual or couple). They don't have to be the original engagement or wedding rings—one can buy a new ring at any time, so it is possible to put some assets into valuable rings; and

■ a burial plot and separate burial fund up to a value of $1,500.

3. TRANSFERRING NON-EXEMPT ASSETS TO AT-HOME SPOUSE

Although transferring non-exempt assets from a nursing facility spouse to an at-home spouse will not initially protect those assets from being counted toward Medicaid eligibility limits (unless they are then transferred to others before Medicaid is applied for, see Section 4, below), such a transfer can save as much as $58,000 if the at-home spouse dies before the nursing facility spouse.

Example: When one spouse is a resident in a nursing facility, Medicaid counts the joint assets of the couple and allows the couple to keep one-half of those combined assets—in some states up to $60,000. But an unmarried nursing facility resident can keep only about $2,000. If the at-home spouse dies, the spouse in the nursing facility becomes an unmarried individual who can only keep $2,000, and the $60,000 the couple had been allowed to keep then automatically goes to pay nursing facility bills.

A couple can avoid losing most of this $60,000 by taking two simple steps. First, the nursing facility spouse transfers the $60,000 into the sole name of the at-home spouse. Then, the at-home spouse makes a will or creates a living trust that leaves the money to the children or to anyone other than the nursing facility spouse. If the at-home spouse dies first, the money goes to the children or other named beneficiary, and not to the nursing facility. (See next section.)

4. TRANSFERRING ASSETS TO CHILDREN OR OTHERS

Some methods of protecting your assets by transferring them to your children or to anyone else other than your spouse, without jeopardizing your Medicaid nursing facility eligibility, have already been mentioned. Here are a couple more points to consider when transferring assets. Remember, though, that transferring assets to children or others means giving up control of those assets. If you need to use the assets, you must depend on the goodwill of your children or anyone else to whom you have transferred them.

TRANSFERS OF EXEMPT ASSETS

Specifically exempt assets—home, car, household goods—may be transferred to children or anyone else even within the 30-month Medicaid no-transfer period. But if assets are exempt, why bother to transfer them? Look back at the Medicaid rules for exempt assets (Chapter 6) and you will see that the exemptions for a married couple with one spouse in a nursing facility are far more generous than for an unmarried individual. But if the at-home spouse dies, a couple's exempt property—home, up to $60,000 in savings, car and household goods of any value—instantly becomes an unmarried person's non-exempt property, and so a source for nursing facility bills. To protect against that, some people transfer title to exempt property as well.

TRANSFERRING NON-EXEMPT PROPERTY THROUGH SPOUSE

As mentioned earlier in this chapter, there is a loophole in the Medicaid transfer rules that allows the transfer of *any* asset from a nursing facility resident to his or her at-home spouse before applying for Medicaid. This permits the spouse either to immediately transfer the assets to children or others, or to set up a living trust.

If the assets are transferred by the at-home spouse before the nursing facility resident applies for Medicaid, they will *not* be counted at all in the couple's joint assets. The problem, however, is that you have given up control over the assets, and are dependent on the goodwill of others to manage them as you would wish. If there is someone in whom you have great trust, this may be a useful asset protection device.

To protect the transferred assets from being counted by Medicaid, a particular sequence of events must be carefully followed:

1. Transferring sole title of assets to the at-home spouse must take place only *after* entering the nursing facility. Because it is possible that the nursing facility spouse may not be legally competent to do this when he or she enters the nursing facility, transfer may only be possible if a durable power of attorney has been previously prepared or a conservator appointed. (See Chapter 8.)

2. Transfer of title must take place *before* the nursing facility resident applies for Medicaid.

3. The at-home spouse also must then transfer title to children or others *before* the nursing facility spouse applies for Medicaid.

If the assets are not transferred by the at-home spouse before the nursing facility spouse applies for Medicaid, the assets will be counted by Medicaid as "joint assets." Even then, it may well be worth transferring sole title to the at-home spouse. Remember that the joint assets a couple is permitted to keep are far greater than for an unmarried individual. Transfer to the at-home spouse at least permits that spouse to leave the assets to children or others in a will, so that if the at-home spouse dies first, the assets will go to loved ones instead of to the nursing facility as part of a suddenly-unmarried resident's assets.

5. PAYMENTS TO CHILDREN FOR SERVICES

Unmarried individuals are at a disadvantage in trying to pass assets to their children or others. Because there is no spouse through whom assets can be transferred, many Medicaid exemption rules do not apply. One way around the 30-month transfer rule is not to transfer assets at all, but instead to pay a child or other person for services performed for you. Such services might be personal care or assistance, transportation, housekeeping, paperwork—almost any reasonable service you would otherwise have to pay someone else to do. Because these are payments rather than transfers, they do not count as transferred assets. However, the Internal Revenue Service and state tax agencies consider these payments as income to the people receiving them, and may require payment of income tax on the amounts received.

As you might guess, Medicaid looks very closely at such arrangements. The services performed must be reasonable and there must be proof they were actually performed. Also, the payments must be reasonable for the services rendered: a thousand dollars for one housecleaning won't pass muster. But payment to an adult child or grandchild for regular housecleaning and maintenance, or for regular transportation, for example, might be acceptable if the amounts paid are within range of the amounts which would have to be paid to a private housecleaning service or for a taxi.

6. IRREVOCABLE TRUST

You have no doubt heard the terms "trust" or "trust fund" and have probably thought it was some complicated legal hocus-pocus for the wealthy. In fact, a trust can be a simple device in which you give up the legal right of ownership over assets but decide on the rules by which they are to be managed, and continue to receive income produced by them. Trusts offer tax benefits and, as discussed below, protection against Medicaid asset rules. If, for example, you have no spouse and no one to whom you want to give immediate control of your assets, but would like to protect your assets for your grandchildren, you could set up an irrevocable trust with your grandchildren as beneficiaries.

If the irrevocable trust is established more than 30 months before you enter a nursing facility or apply for Medicaid, its assets do not count in determining your eligibility for Medicaid. Trust assets will be used in accordance with the rules you set up for the trustee, for the benefit of the beneficiaries. But remember, for the trust to be effective in protecting the assets from nursing facility costs, it must be "irrevocable." That means that once the assets are put in the trust, they are out of your control forever.

You will probably need help from an attorney to set up a trust, since fixing the amount of control you can maintain over the assets may require the skills of a specialist. Also, the tax consequences for both the person setting up the trust and the beneficiaries should be considered before any trust is created.

7. MEDICAID AND DIVORCE

It may seem strange to think of divorce in connection with long-term care, but the unfortunate effect of the Medicaid income and assets limits has been to force more than a few couples to divorce for solely economic reasons. If all other methods for transferring or otherwise protecting assets are unavailable, or the eligibility problem is with continuing income, you may at least want to consider the unpleasant alternative of divorce. Remember, though, that all that is required to change Medicaid status is the formal, legal divorce. A couple need not stop living together or in any other way change their relationship. In fact, no one has to be told about the divorce except Medicaid.

This situation often arises when a couple must choose between entering a nursing facility and being covered by Medicaid, or remaining home without coverage. About thirty states have no income eligibility levels for Medicaid coverage of residential nursing facility care; the other states have income levels of $700 to $1,100 per month for eligibility, but allow the at-home spouse to keep all income in his or her name. And all states allow the at-home spouse of a nursing facility resident to keep between $12,000 and $60,000 in savings or other assets.

For non-nursing facility care, on the other hand, all states have severe limits on the amount of income and assets a couple can have and still qualify for Medicaid coverage. A couple may thus be forced to choose between getting care at home and being disqualified from Medicare, or getting divorced. A divorce permits the working spouse to keep all of his or her income without disqualifying the other spouse and allows the protection of at least half of the couple's assets without limit. The spouse (now ex-spouse) needing care can then remain at home and receive Medicaid-covered home care.

A couple may face the same difficult choice about whether to end their marriage for economic reasons even when one spouse is already in a nursing facility. If they live in a state with income eligibility limits for nursing facility couples and the at-home spouse continues to work and make more than the allowable income, that would disqualify the nursing facility spouse from coverage. Similarly, if a couple has considerably more in savings and other non-exempt assets than the Medicaid rules of their state would permit them to keep, a divorce settlement that gives more assets to the at-home spouse than Medicaid would have allowed the couple to keep may be a way of holding on to savings.

These are all matters that depend, however, on both the specific Medicaid rules and divorce laws of your state. If divorce seems like the best last resort for you, consult a lawyer who is familiar both with divorce law and with Medicaid.

PROTECTING AN ELDER'S HEALTH CARE AND BUSINESS CHOICES

PROTECTING AN ELDER'S HEALTH CARE AND BUSINESS CHOICES

One of the difficult truths of aging is that as physical and mental capabilities diminish, many elders must depend on others to take care of life's business for them. A number of legal and practical roadblocks can complicate this shifting of responsibility, however. And when an elder becomes incapable of making decisions, there can be enormous problems not only in trying to get business affairs accomplished, but also in handling them exactly as the elder would wish. Finally, taking care of an elder's business is also difficult because it signals the need to face the process of dying and the aftermath of death.

This chapter discusses:

- how to protect the rights, dignity and wishes of an elder who is no longer competent to make decisions, including exceedingly difficult choices about medical interventions and the right to die; and

- how to protect an elder in financial transactions if the elder becomes incapable of handling his or her own affairs.

The increasing use of life-sustaining medical machines over the last decades has raised a fear in many of us that our lives may be artificially prolonged against our wishes. The "right to die" with dignity, and without the tremendous agony and expense for family caused by artificial life-prolonging, has been addressed in many states by "medical directive laws." These laws, although different in scope and method, all authorize some form of written document—a power of attorney for health care, a living will, or both—by which people can direct physicians and hospitals concerning the use of life-prolonging medical technologies.

The purpose of both a living will and a durable power of attorney for health care decisions, broadly referred to as "medical directives," is to ensure that your health care wishes are carried out if you become mentally or physically unable to express yourself. Both legal devices allow you to make your wishes known to a treating physician or to a trusted friend or family member who will then be able to direct your medical care on your behalf. Both can help relieve family members from having to make agonizing decisions about a loved one's medical treatment. The documents act as an enduring directive of your wishes if you become incapacitated and your loved ones—your spouse, companion, parents, siblings or children—have differing ideas on what care you should receive. Also, doctors and hospitals have their own rules and beliefs about what is proper medical treatment, and even if your family knows your wishes and tries to have them granted, the medical personnel would not necessarily be bound to follow them without a valid document signed by you.

A. DURABLE POWERS OF ATTORNEY

A power of attorney is a document in which one person (the "principal") gives authority to another to act if he or she becomes unable to act—to ensure wishes for medical treatment are carried out, to make business decisions, spend or receive money, or take other actions in the principal's best interest. The person appointed is called an "attorney-in-fact"—a potentially confusing term since the person does *not* have to be an attorney at law. The best choice for an attorney-in-fact is usually a family member or trusted friend—someone with knowledge and respect for your personal and financial wishes.

The principal can create a power of attorney for a definite or indefinite period of time, for specific or very broad decision-making, effective immediately or at some future time. As long as the principal remains legally competent, he or she may change or end the power of attorney at any time, and can specify that the attorney-in-fact's powers take effect only when the principal can no longer act.

The principal must be legally competent to create or modify a power of attorney. But a "durable" power of attorney remains in effect even when the principal becomes legally incompetent. Thus, a durable power of attorney is a way to make sure that someone of your choice will manage your affairs and make crucial decisions about your comfort, health and even your life if you become incapacitated.

1. DURABLE POWER OF ATTORNEY FOR HEALTH CARE

The durable power of attorney for health care authorizes someone else to act in your behalf if you become incapacitated. Some durable powers of attorney go into effect as soon as you sign them.

But if you do not want to share authority while you are still competent to make decisions yourself, you can use a "springing" durable power of attorney, which has no effect unless and until you become legally incompetent, when it "springs" into use. You can even include the stipulation that your physician must certify in writing that you are incompetent before the power of attorney can become effective.

In many states, you can tailor a durable power of attorney to your own needs, combining specific instructions about life support systems and medical care with authority to make financial and other personal decisions. Or, as is required in a few states, you can create a separate power of attorney for medical care, which appoints an individual attorney-in-fact to handle your health care decisions.

One power of attorney document granting authority to make medical decisions is enough, since having more could cause confusion. But, of course, you can revoke a power of attorney and create a new one if you wish to change your attorney-in-fact or your health care choices.

There are basically three approaches to medical care you can take with a durable power of attorney:

- You can direct that life support systems be used;
- You can direct that life support systems *not* be used after diagnosis of a fatal, incurable or irreversible condition; or
- You can leave the decision regarding the use of life support to your appointed attorney-in-fact.

Within these general categories, you can include specific authorizations to the attorney-in-fact, such as:

- to give, withhold or withdraw consent to medical or surgical procedures;
- to consent to appropriate care for the end of life—including procedures for pain relief;
- to hire and fire medical personnel;

- to have access to medical records and other personal information;
- to get any court authorization required to obtain or withhold medical treatment (which might be required if a hospital or physician for some reason does not honor the authority of the power of attorney itself); and
- to spend or withhold money necessary to carry out medical treatment.

Currently, not all states have laws that officially authorize durable powers of attorney for medical care. But the fact that a state does not specifically authorize it does not necessarily mean that a durable power of attorney would not be honored. In fact, there is a strong legal trend to recognize them everywhere. This makes sense when you realize a durable power of attorney is often the only and best evidence a doctor or court has regarding a person's wishes for their own care.

Among those states which specifically authorize them, the rules vary as to the forms required, when the power can go into effect and whether an attorney-in-fact can *refuse* medical treatment or merely *consent* to it. (See the following list of states that have medical directive laws.) Nevertheless, limits on, or unknowns about, the effectiveness of a power of attorney in many states make it advisable that you also prepare a living will for added protection. (See Section B.)

2. DURABLE POWER OF ATTORNEY FOR FINANCIAL MANAGEMENT

As mentioned above, you can also draw up a specific type of durable power of attorney authorizing the attorney-in-fact to manage your financial matters. For older people especially, a durable power of attorney for financial management provides peace of mind that their money and property will be managed by a trusted person with no need for a court-appointed guardian or conservator—procedures that are cumbersome, expensive and public—should they be stricken by a debilitating disease or need to face an operation. Older people can tailor a durable power of attorney to their practical needs—authorizing an attorney-in-fact to take care of financial matters ranging from buying holiday gifts for others to the more mundane: paying bills, making bank deposits, handling insurance and Social Security paperwork, selling a home or other property.

The success of any power of attorney arrangement depends upon the trust between you and your attorney-in-fact. But when you know in advance what specific actions you do and do not want an attorney-in-fact to take with your money or other property, those should be written into the document as specific limits on the attorney-in-fact's authority. And some people name more than one attorney-in-fact in the same power of attorney document, with a provision that both must agree on any transaction involving property over a certain amount.[1]

POWERS OF ATTORNEY AND MEDICAID

As explained in Chapter 7, there are a number of ways to protect your assets from the reach of a nursing facility while still qualifying for Medicaid. Several of these methods, however, might require a transfer of assets after you are no longer capable of doing so. If you create a limited power of attorney, make sure it would permit the attorney-in-fact to make transactions necessary to protect your assets if you are incapacitated, such as the power to transfer your property to a spouse, children or other specifically-named people.

POWERS OF ATTORNEY AND LIVING TRUSTS

Even if you already have a revocable living trust and as part of this document have provided for property management should you become incapacitated, it may be a good idea to have a durable power of attorney as well. (See the discussion of living trusts in Chapter 9.) A living trust covers only property already in the trust at the time you become unable to make decisions. The trustee will have no authority over property received after that—Social Security, pension benefits, any other income or assets—but an attorney-in-fact designated in a durable power of attorney will. Also, a living trust can only deal with financial matters. It cannot cover health care decisions—one of the important uses of a power of attorney.

---

[1]For step-by-step assistance and the forms required to prepare a power of attorney, see *The Power of Attorney Book* by Denis Clifford (Nolo Press).

B. LIVING WILLS

A living will is not a will at all, but a document stating a person's decision to refuse medical treatment, particularly artificial life-support. Sometimes called a Directive to Physicians or Advanced Directive, a living will is presented directly to a doctor, hospital or other medical provider. It becomes part of a patient's official medical record, legally binding the physician or hospital to follow the patient's wishes.

Most states permit living wills, although the laws vary from state to state. Some of the variables are:

- Each state requires you to use its own form and will not recognize a living will prepared on a different form. (See, How to Obtain the Right Form, below.)

- Some states permit a living will to name another person—a "proxy"—who can make medical decisions if you are incapacitated. This type of living will is similar to a durable power of attorney for health care.

- Unlike a power of attorney, some states require that a living will be signed only *after* a patient has been diagnosed with a terminal condition. Others have time limits within which the paperwork must be completed. These provisions do not protect against an accident or sudden onset of an incapacitating terminal condition—a good reason to prepare a durable power of attorney for health care as well as a living will.

- In some states, a living will expires periodically and must be signed and witnessed again—typically, every five years.

A possible problem with living wills is that some are not specific enough for a doctor to figure out which medical treatments are prohibited and which are not. To take care of this, it is best to name the treatments you know you do not want—artificial feeding, mechanical breathing machine, for example. It is also best to name a proxy to decide on other treatments not specifically mentioned in the living will.

Note on Preparing Two Documents: As mentioned, it is often an excellent precaution to have both a living will and a durable power of attorney for health care. You can prepare both forms yourself (see below) and there is little or no cost. If you do prepare both, make sure they are consistent. Your attorney-in-fact for health care should be the same person as the proxy named in your living will and the language used to describe medical treatment you do not want should be the same in both documents.

■ _____

SOME TIPS ON MEDICAL DIRECTIVES

- Do *not* appoint your physician as your proxy or attorney-in-fact. Your physician can advise, but should not be left to make final medical decisions for you.
- Show your doctor your proposed medical directive. If your doctor disagrees with any part of it, or has suggestions, discuss it until you are certain the doctor will follow what you finally decide upon. If the doctor will not agree to follow the directive, consider changing doctors.
- Consider appointing a second person as back-up proxy or attorney-in-fact to act if the first person is unable or unwilling to act for you. Make sure the second person gets a copy of all relevant documents.
- Make several copies of your living will or durable power of attorney and give a signed copy to several family members, your doctor, lawyer or clergy. Each *signed* copy is legally the same as an "original" document. If you make any changes later, remember to update each document.
- Re-date and re-sign your living will at least once a year.

■

STATES WITH MEDICAL DIRECTIVE LAWS

Living Wills

Alabama	Minnesota
Alaska	Mississippi
Arizona	Missouri
Arkansas	Montana
California	Nevada
Colorado	New Hampshire
Connecticut	New Mexico
Delaware	North Carolina
District of Columbia	North Dakota
Florida	Oklahoma
Georgia	Oregon
Hawaii	South Carolina
Idaho	Tennessee
Illinois	Texas
Indiana	Utah
Iowa	Vermont
Kansas	Virginia
Kentucky	Washington
Louisiana	West Virginia
Maine	Wisconsin
Maryland	Wyoming

Power of Attorney for Health Care

Alaska	North Carolina*
California	Pennsylvania*
Colorado*	Rhode Island
District of Columbia	South Dakota
Idaho	Texas
Illinois	Utah
Maine	Vermont
New Mexico	Washington
Maryland	West Virginia
Nevada	

*State authorizes an attorney-in-fact to consent to medical treatment but does not specify whether he or she can refuse it.

C. HOW TO OBTAIN THE RIGHT FORM FOR A MEDICAL DIRECTIVE

In most instances, you do not need to consult a lawyer to prepare either a living will or a durable power of attorney for health care. You may also be able to find the forms required in your state by calling the Senior Referral and Information number in the white pages of the telephone directory.

For assistance and information, contact the national non-profit organization Society for the Right to Die, one of the oldest patients' advocacy groups in the country. The Society welcomes donations, but provides free information on your state's current laws on both living wills and durable powers of attorney for health care, including current forms. Send your request with a stamped, self-addressed envelope to:

Society for the Right to Die
250 West 57th Street
New York, NY 10107
(212) 246-6973

Also, all the necessary forms and instructions required to complete durable powers of attorney—both for health care and financial management—are available in:

The Power of Attorney Book
by Denis Clifford
3rd National Edition
Nolo Press
$19.95

D. GUARDIANSHIPS AND CONSERVATORSHIPS

Much of the advice so far in this chapter may not apply to you if the elder you are concerned about is already incapacitated and unable to make decisions. At that point, the elder can no longer enter into legal documents and arrangements or delegate responsibility for decisions to others. Yet there is a danger that without prior legal arrangements such as a durable power of attorney or living trust, financial institutions, government agencies, health care providers and bureaucrats of every variety will either refuse to take action regarding the elder's affairs, or will take actions without regard for your wishes or for what you know are the elder's wishes.

In this situation, you may have to go to court to ask a judge to appoint you or another friend or relative to act on the elder's behalf. There are procedures in every state to do this. Some states have only one legal category, usually called guardianship, while others have a second category, usually called conservatorship and often limited to financial matters.

In general guardianship proceedings, the legal question is whether or not the elder has become "incompetent" to handle any of his or her own affairs. In about half the states, this requires that medical evidence of incompetence be presented to the court. In more limited proceedings to establish a financial conservatorship or guardianship only (see below), the court can act if it finds that the elder is unable to handle financial affairs even though not completely legally incompetent.

In conservatorship or guardianship proceedings, an elder has a right to appear in court with an attorney and to consent or object to all proposed authority. In many states, if the elder does not have an attorney, the court may appoint one. Similarly, any change in the conservator or guardian's authority requires an additional court order to which the elder can consent or object. The conservator or guardian is held responsible for mismanagement of the elder's property.

In some states, it is possible to handle conservatorship proceedings without the assistance of a lawyer if no one challenges the need for the conservatorship and its scope. More complicated guardianship procedures, however, do require the assistance of a lawyer, particularly if the elder or anyone else does not agree that the guardianship is needed or that the person seeking to be guardian is not the right person for the job.

1. FINANCIAL CONSERVATORSHIP OR GUARDIANSHIP

A conservator or guardian can be appointed by a court solely to protect an elder's property (savings, real estate, investments). He or she can also conduct daily financial affairs (such as paying bills) or arrange for services when the elder is unable to do so. This type of limited management assistance is appropriate when the elder is still capable of caring for himself or herself, but because of disorientation or disability is unable to carry out personal business affairs efficiently. In this situation, the conservator or guardian does *not* have power over the elder's personal conduct, but has authority over financial or other affairs as the court orders.

An advantage of a limited conservatorship or guardianship is that it leaves an elder free to make many important decisions independently: where to live, with whom to associate, what medical care to receive, how to handle property. Nonetheless, it is still a court process in which a judge makes a ruling, occasionally against the elder's will, that gives another person authority over some parts of his or her life. It is therefore a procedure to be used only if voluntary procedures such as a durable power of attorney are no longer possible.

2. FULL GUARDIANSHIP

Full guardianship is an extreme measure that severely restricts the legal rights of an elder based on a court's finding of legal "incompetence." It reduces one's legal status to that of a minor, with no control over one's own money or property, decisions about medical care or institutionalization. A person under guardianship even loses the right to vote.

If an elder retains some degree of orientation and capability, a legal finding by a court that he or she is "incompetent" can be emotionally devastating and, in fact, self-fulfilling. The person deemed legally incompetent may well give up the will to care for himself or herself and become much less competent than before. Obviously, full guardianship is a very serious step, to be taken when a person's mental condition leaves no other choice such as a durable power of attorney.

■

CONSERVATORSHIPS, GUARDIANSHIPS AND MEDICAID

A conservator or guardian is under a legal obligation to act only in the best interests of the elder. As has been discussed over the last three chapters, there are times when the best interests of the elder with respect to qualifying for Medicaid may involve transferring assets to a spouse, child or other person. Taken at face value, giving away someone's property does not appear to be in that person's best interests. Therefore, before a conservator or guardian transfers an elder's property for Medicaid purposes, it is advisable to go to court, explain the proposed transfer and get the court's approval.

ESTATE PLANNING: PROTECTING AN ELDER'S MONEY AND PROPERTY

ESTATE PLANNING: PROTECTING AN ELDER'S MONEY AND PROPERTY

"Estate planning" refers to actions you can take while living to determine what happens to your property when you die. It includes:

- deciding who will get your property when you die;
- setting up procedures and devices to make sure your property passes to others free from probate, or that your estate owes the least amount possible in probate fees;
- particularly if your estate is a large one, setting up ways to pass your property to others while reducing or avoiding taxes; and
- setting up management for property you want to go to others who might need outside help in managing it—including minors, an older or unhealthy spouse or companion or a person with tendencies to being a spendthrift or substance abuser.

Some people leave estate planning to lawyers, although the basic steps are easy enough to do yourself if you are willing to spend some time wading through rules and making some difficult decisions. The discussion in this chapter is by no means a comprehensive guide to estate planning, but it should help alert you to some of your options.

■

NOLO PRESS ESTATE PLANNING RESOURCES

Should your interest be piqued enough to learn in more detail what estate planning steps you can take on your own, Nolo Press publishes several comprehensive resources to help you. All of them are good in every state but Louisiana:

- *Plan Your Estate: Wills, Probate Avoidance, Trusts & Taxes* by Denis Clifford. This book covers all aspects of basic estate planning and is especially suited to those whose estates are worth $1 million or less.

- *WillMaker* by Nolo and Legisoft. This computer software available for Macintosh and IBM compatible computers allows you to create your own basic will, including trusts that allow you to name a responsible adult to manage property on behalf of children. The accompanying manual provides explanations and examples to guide you.
- *Nolo's Simple Will Book* by Denis Clifford. This book includes all the instructions and forms you need to draft a legally valid will—one that can be tailored to include naming a guardian and a property manager for minor children.

A. THE BASIC NEED: A WILL

Despite their own best interests, and often despite their own best intentions, many people do not have a will—the legal document that directs how to parcel out a person's property after death. And others may have a will drawn up so long ago that it no longer accurately reflects the will-maker's wishes, assets or family circumstances.

If you die without leaving a will, you are said to die "intestate." Your property will then be distributed to your spouse, children or other relatives if you have no spouse or children, according to the statutory formula or "intestate succession laws" in your state.

Even if you opt to transfer your property to others using other techniques such as a probate-avoiding living trust, preparing a simple will is an essential first step to planning any estate. In a will, not only do you spell out who you want to get your property, you can also name a personal representative (executor) to round up and distribute that property and to wind up your business and financial affairs after your death. A will also provides an opportunity for you to name a personal guardian for your own minor children and to name someone to manage property for any minor or young adult child to whom you leave property—until they reach an age you believe they will be capable of managing it alone.

Finally, because a living trust only works to dispose of property transferred by the trust, a will is necessary to take care of other property—especially property you acquire shortly before death.

Note that a "living will," discussed in Chapter 8, is something completely different from the kind of will discussed here. Living wills let you express your wishes about medical treatment in case you become ill or incapacitated; they are not devices to transfer property after death.

B. AVOIDING PROBATE

Probate is the legal process by which a person's property, called an "estate," is distributed after death. It involves filing a will, if there is one, with the local probate court; identifying and appraising all the person's property; and paying debts and estate taxes and distributing what's left of the property according to the instructions in the will or according to state law if there is no will—all with the approval of the court. Except for small estates in the wide range of $5,000 to $60,000, depending on the state, and, in some states, for property left from one spouse to the other, all property left by a will must go through probate.

Fees for lawyers, appraisers, accountants and the probate court, which often total 5% to 7% or more of the value of the deceased person's estate, reduce the property that ultimately goes to the beneficiaries.

Another problem is that probate usually takes nine to eighteen months to complete and requires time and effort by the executor or administrator who is responsible for collecting and then distributing the estate property. Because of the cost and inconvenience of probate, many people arrange for distribution of their property through legal devices that avoid probate. Several of these methods—joint tenancy, pay-on death accounts, life insurance, living trusts and retirement accounts—are discussed briefly below, with special attention to their implications for estate planning for older people.

1. JOINT TENANCY

Joint tenancy is one of the most popular probate avoidance devices. Unfortunately, for older property owners, it is often fraught with unforeseen difficulties. Still, for many, joint tenancy is an easy way to prepare to handle simple finances—maintaining bank accounts, paying household bills—when the elder is no longer capable of doing so.[1]

In a joint tenancy, two or more people own the same property equally. Joint tenancy carries with it the "right of survivorship." This means that when one joint tenant dies, his or her share of the joint tenancy property automatically passes to, and becomes owned by, the surviving joint tenants. They need not go through probate or other legal gyrations to get full ownership of the property.

Joint tenancy is particularly useful as a management device for relatively small assets such as joint bank accounts. And, for older people, it may offer some convenience. If an elder becomes ill and is unable to get to the bank or becomes unable to manage his or her affairs, for example, a joint tenant on the account can take care of the finances without having to go through complicated bank or court procedures.

In most states, joint tenancy is easy to set up and can be done without an attorney, and without cost, by filling out a simple form available at the bank, stock brokerage or other financial institution that holds the assets.

Because each joint tenant has equal access to funds, there is always the danger that one joint tenant will misuse them, especially if large amounts are involved. Accordingly, joint tenancy is advisable only when there is complete trust between joint tenants. Older people, many of whom are vulnerable to those eager to defraud them of their assets, should be on the look-out for those who attempt to entrap them into suddenly changing ownership of their property.

In some states, you can protect against the risk of misuse by opening a joint tenancy bank account that requires the signatures of *both* joint tenants before withdrawals can be made. The problem with this arrangement, though, is that much of the convenience of joint tenancy is lost. If both signatures are required, joint tenancy funds would not be easily available if the elder becomes incapacitated.

Because property held in joint tenancy passes automatically at death, it also can be a useful probate avoidance tool for couples and

---

[1]Somewhat different rules apply to joint tenancy property in different states and it goes by different names—"tenancy by the entirety" for joint tenant married couples in some states; other states require the use of the term "right of survivorship."

other long-term co-owners of property who want the survivors to get their share. However, transferring solely-owned property into joint tenancy is not usually the best method to avoid probate.

First, the IRS often considers a transfer of solely-owned property into joint tenancy to be a taxable gift. If the new joint tenant did not pay full market value for his or her share, the transaction is legally considered to be a gift. With real estate, in particular, the gift is considered to be legally made when the new joint tenant is listed on the deed and it is recorded with the county land records office. If the value of the gift exceeds $10,000, a federal gift tax return must be filed by the giver of the gift. The exception is that money placed in a joint bank account is not a gift until the other person removes some of the money.

When the giver dies, the full market value of the real estate, as of the giver's death, is included in the giver's taxable estate, even though ta half-interest was already given away during the giver's life. The giver's estate receives a tax credit for the gift tax previously assessed.

Using a living trust to achieve this goal avoids possibles problems with a gift tax return because there is no transfer until the original owner dies. However, transferring solely-owned property into joint tenancy can be useful as a last minute probate avoidance device, when death is imminent, if no living trust has been prepared and there is not sufficient time to prepare one.

Second, placing property in joint tenancy does not protect an asset in the face of Medicaid eligibility rules. As discussed in Chapter 6, these rules force an elder to spend most of his or her assets before Medicaid will begin to pay anything for a nursing facility or long-term care. But if assets are large enough, it makes good sense to take steps other than joint tenancy to protect them from these Medicaid rules. (See Chapter 7 for a detailed discussion of how to protect assets.)

2. PAY-ON-DEATH ACCOUNTS

Most banks and savings institutions let depositors name someone to receive the contents of an account free of probate at the depositor's death. The depositor keeps sole control of the account during his or her lifetime, but whatever is in the account then passes to the beneficiary upon the depositor's death. Often called pay-on-death accounts or informal trusts, they provide a simple way of passing on money without having it go through probate. Some types of federal securities allso allow the owner to make a pay-on-death designation.

However, this arrangement is not helpful if the depositor becomes incompetent, since no one else has access to that account during the depositor's lifetime. A durable power of attorney naming another person to handle financial matters can, however, be used to give him or her legal access to the account in the event the depositor becomes incompetent. (See the discussion of durable powers of attorney in Chapter 8.)

3. LIFE INSURANCE

Life insurance is another way to transfer money with no need for probate. This is because you name the beneficiary of the policy in the policy itself, and not in your will. The only time the property will be subject to probate is if you name your estate as the beneficiary on the policy. That set-up is made occasionally if the estate will need immediate cash to pay debts and taxes, but it is fairly uncommon. (See Section C1 for a discussion of making a gift of life insurance while you are alive to save on estate taxes.)

4. PENSION PLANS OR RETIREMENT ACCOUNTS

Retirement accounts such as IRAs and Keogh Accounts were not originally intended to be probate avoidance devices, but they can easily be used that way. All you do is name a beneficiary to receive the funds still in your pension plan or retirement account at your death, and the funds will not pass through probate.

After you reach age 70, however, federal law requires you to withdraw a minimum amount every year or face a monetary penalty. The amount you must withdraw is recomputed every year, based on your life expectancy.

5. LIVING TRUSTS

A living trust is the safest and most comprehensive way to avoid probate. A trust is a legal entity, created by a document. It has the legal capacity to own property. Money or other property owned by a trust may be spent only according to the terms of the document that established the trust.

Trust assets are managed by someone called the "trustee," appointed by the person who sets up the trust, who is called the "trustor" or "settlor." Legally, a trustee can be any competent adult. For most living trusts, however, the trustor appoints himself or herself as trustee. This allows the elder who sets up the trust to keep full control over the trust property—and avoid probate, too.

The trust document also names a successor trustee to take over if the elder becomes incapacitated or dies. The trustee or successor trustee must administer the trust according to the elder's written trust instructions, which can be changed or revoked at any time, as long as the elder is competent. Upon the elder's death, the successor trustee distributes the assets according to the elder's trust instructions. This process functions very much like a will but without probate.

Example: Tony wants to leave his valuable painting collection to his son and his home to his daughter, but wants to have and enjoy all the paintings and to continue to live in his home during his own lifetime. He also does not want the value of his extensive collection and real property—which are worth nearly $1 million dollars combined—to be included in his probate estate when he dies. Tony takes care of all these concerns by establishing a living trust for the paintings, naming himself trustee while he lives, with his son the beneficiary of the paintings and his daughter of the house. He names his trusted friend Mavis as successor trustee. When Tony dies, Mavis will transfer the painting collection and house to his children outside of probate.

There are a number of advantages to a revocable living trust. While alive, the trustor retains complete control over the assets. And instructions to a trustee can be as specific or as general as the elder wants. Because the trust can be controlled by the elder—either as trustee, by changing trust instructions, or by adding or subtracting trust assets—there is no risk of misuse of the funds as there is with a joint tenancy, which actually makes the eventual inheritor a co-owner of the property. Trust assets are also protected in the case of incapacity, because the successor trustee is normally empowered to handle them according to instructions. At death, assets are distributed to inheritors free of probate.

In many situations, simple living trusts can be set up without the use of an attorney and administered by a friend or relative as trustee.[2] More complicated living trusts, however, may require an attorney to establish and to make later changes, and a bank or attorney to act as trustee.

REVOCABLE LIVING TRUSTS AND MEDICAID

If a living trust is revocable, its assets are *not* exempt from Medicaid eligibility limits. However, it is possible to create a revocable living trust with specific instructions to the trustee to transfer assets in a way that will get the most Medicaid eligibility and require the least in payment to a nursing facility. Those instructions must be very carefully written to take advantage of the asset protection methods which may be available to you as described in Chapter 7.

---

[2]The forms and instructions you need to set up a living trust on your own are contained in *Plan Your Estate* by Denis Clifford (Nolo Press).

C. SAVING ON ESTATE TAXES

If you, or you and your spouse have a combined estate worth less than $600,000, and you have not already given away large amounts of property, you will not likely be affected by federal estate tax concerns. However, if your estate, or the combined estate of you and your spouse exceeds $600,000, you face a hefty estate tax liability. Marginal tax rates begin at 37% for the first non-exempt dollar over $600,000 and go up fairly rapidly from there.

It is important to understand that the federal government taxes estates and gifts made during life at the same rate. In setting up that system, Congress reasoned that if only gifts made at death were taxed, everyone would simply give as much property as they could during their lives. Tax avoidance would become the norm instead of the aim. However, (as discussed in Section 2 below), yearly gifts of less than $10,000 per recipient are completely exempt from federal gift tax.

Fortunately, in addition to the basic $600,000 exemption, there are several other important estate tax exemptions. The most significant exemption is for property left to a surviving spouse. Quite simply, all property left to a surviving spouse is exempt from federal estate taxes. But caution: For larger estates, the fact that no federal estate tax is assessed may lead to a substantial tax liability when the second spouse dies. (See Section C1 for a discussion of how a marital trust can help deal with this.)

The other main exemptions from estate tax are:
- the expenses of a last illness;
- burial costs;
- probate fees and expenses;
- certain debts, including a credit for state death taxes and death taxes imposed by foreign countries on property the deceased person owned there; and
- all tax-deductible charitable gifts made in a will.

1. MARITAL TRUSTS

A type of trust called a marital life estate trust, which can be established under a will as a testamentary trust, or as part of a living trust, is one of the simplest ways to provide for management of funds with the added advantage, in some circumstances, of saving money on estate taxes. With a marital life estate trust, the elder completely controls the use of the assets during his or her lifetime. Upon the elder's death, the assets in the trust are administered by a trustee named by the elder under the terms specified in the will.

A marital trust is especially advisable for an elderly couple who has combined assets of over $600,000—the normal threshold at which federal estate taxes must be paid. If they each leave all their property to each other, with the surviving spouse then leaving the entire estate to other inheritors (such as their children), the total estate taxes will be based on all non-exempt property worth over $600,000. The way a marital trust can save on taxes is that it allows each member of the couple to use his or her entire $600,000 estate tax exemption. It prevents the surviving spouse from ending up with all the property belonging to both spouses, and assuming this is more than $600,000, saves the survivor's estate a hefty estate tax liability.

A marital trust works like this: Income from trust property, and in some cases the property itself, is left for the use of the surviving spouse during the other's lifetime, but the survivor never actually becomes the legal owner of the property. Since legal ownership bypasses the surviving spouse, the obligation of that spouse's estate to pay estate tax on the money received from the first spouse to die is also bypassed.

2. GIFTS

An excellent way to reduce your estate tax liability is to reduce the size of your estate by giving property to the same people you would ultimately like to leave it to anyway. Because gifts are taxed at the same rate as money left in an estate, savings can be realized by making a number of small gifts—as many as you want to and can afford to give—that are less than the annual $10,000 gift tax exemption. Here are the rules:

- You can give away property in amounts of $10,000 or less per person or organization per year, absolutely tax-free.
- A couple can give $20,000 a year tax-free to one person and $40,000 to another couple.
- This strategy can be repeated year after year. So giving gifts to reduce estate tax liability works well for people who have enough property so that they can afford to be generous. It's a particularly good strategy for reasonably affluent people who have several children, grandchildren or other objects of affection. If these children are married and the couple wishes to include spouses and children in their gift-giving program, these amounts can be greatly increased.

Example: Albert, whose estate is worth $1,000,000, gives $400,000 to children and grandchildren over five years. His estate tax liability is reduced from nearly $250,000 to 0.

■
_____

GIFTS OF INSURANCE

The proceeds of life insurance are included in your estate for federal estate tax purposes if you own the policy. If you think your estate will be liable for federal estate taxes—which usually means it must be worth more than $600,000 at your death, you can reduce the tax bill by transferring ownership of the policy before your death. This is a particularly good strategy because gift tax liability is imposed on the cash value of the policy at the time it is given, which is likely to be substantially less than its pay-off value at death. Once you have transferred ownership of the policy, the proceeds will not be counted as part of your taxable estate.

To satisfy the Internal Revenue Service that you have authentically transferred ownership of a life insurance policy, you must verify that you have given up total interest in the policy; you cannot keep the right to name beneficiaries, cancel coverage, borrow against the policy or make payments on it.

One final twist: You must transfer ownership of the policy—usually by completing a few simple forms you can get from your insurance company—*at least three years before your death*, or the IRS will count it as part of your taxable estate.

In making $10,000 annual gifts, it is a particularly good idea to give property that is likely to go up in value in the future. Otherwise, the increase in value would add to the net worth of the elder's estate if it goes over the $600,000 untaxed limit.

3. STATE DEATH TAXES

About half the states impose death taxes on:

- all real estate owned in the state, no matter where the deceased person lived, and
- all other property of residents of the state, no matter where the property is located.

Home is where the tax is. Your taxability will be assessed in the state deemed your "legal residence." To establish a legal residence in a particular state, register all vehicles there, keep bank accounts there and vote in that state.

If you live in a state that does not impose death taxes and you do not own real property in a state that imposes them, they need be of no concern to you. But if you spend different parts of the year in more than one state, it will allow your inheritors to take your personal property free of state inheritance tax if you establish your permanent legal residence in a state that does not have the taxes.

■

STATES THAT HAVE EFFECTIVELY ABOLISHED
STATE DEATH TAXES INCLUDE: [3]

Alabama	Hawaii	Oregon
Alaska	Illinois	Texas
Arizona	Maine	Utah
Arkansas	Minnesota	Vermont
California	Missouri	Virginia
Colorado	Nevada	West Virginia
District of Columbia	New Mexico	Washington
Florida	North Dakota	Wyoming
Georgia		

Example: Harry and Margot, an elderly married couple, spend their winters in Florida and summers in New York. Florida has no death taxes. New York imposes comparatively stiff estate taxes—with rates ranging from 2% for 50,000 or less to 21% for $10,100,000 or more. It probably makes good sense for Harry and Margot to make Florida their legal residence. To do this, they should register to vote in Florida and conduct as many business transactions there as possible—for example, using Florida banks and registering vehicles in Florida. It might also make sense for them to sell any real property located in New York and simply rent when they are in that state.

D. MANAGING PROPERTY

Ongoing trusts can be used to provide for the management and control of property when a person doesn't want to turn that property over to the beneficiary outright. Some beneficiaries, such as minors or people who have been declared legally incompetent, are not permitted to control substantial amounts of property on their own. Or the beneficiary may be seriously disabled, a spendthrift or have drug or

---

[3]Many of these states impose an inheritance tax in theory. However, the maximum amount of the state death tax is equal to the maximum amount for state taxes allowed under federal estate tax law. As a result, an estate pays no more tax than it would have if the state levied no inheritance tax.

alcohol abuse problems—all situations that may make it feasible for another person to be appointed property manager through a trust with the power to dole out money to the spendthrift on a periodic basis.

Property management trusts are a good option for an older person who wishes to pass property to someone who fits into one of these categories. With managerial trusts, it is particularly important to select a responsible trustee, someone who is attuned to the beneficiaries' needs. This is because the trustee will have an ongoing relationship with the beneficiaries and will also have important decisions to make, such as how to invest trust money and whether to expend part of the trust principal to meet special needs of the beneficiary.

1. SPECIAL CONCERNS FOR SUBSEQUENT MARRIAGES

People who marry more than once may face problems reconciling their desires for their present spouse and family with their wishes to be sure to pass property to the children from their prior marriages. Individual situations vary drastically, and you must carefully evaluate your desires to tailor your legal set-up to your situation.

Example: Gertrude, in her 70s, is wealthy and has three grown children. She remarries Ted, also in his 70s. Ted has very little property and has two children from a prior marriage who Gertrude feels are both spoiled and ungrateful. As she plans her estate, Gertrude realizes that she wants to allow Ted to remain in the house if she dies before he does, but does not want him to be able to lease the property to her pushy kids. Understandably, Gertrude's own children share her concerns.

Gertrude decides to give some of her property outright to her children. She also decides to create a trust for the house and to leave enough money in that trust to pay for the mortgage and upkeep on the house. The trust will specify that Ted has the right to live in the house for his lifetime, with the house to go to Gertrude's kids at Ted's death.

COMPARISON OF ASSET PROTECTION DEVICES

	Elder retains control of assets	Avoids probate	Can be set up easily without an attorney	Automatic protection of assets under Medicaid	Permits transfer of assets to protect re Medicaid	Possible tax benefits	Protection if elder becomes incompetent	Can be revoked by elder
Will	yes	no	yes	no	yes	yes	no	yes
Joint Tenancy	shared control	yes	yes	no	yes	yes	no	no
Pay-on-Death Bank Account	yes	yes	yes	no	no	no	no	yes
Trust under Will	yes	yes	no	maybe[1]	yes[2]	yes	no	yes or no[3]
Revocable Living Trust	yes	yes	yes	no	yes	yes	yes	yes
Durable Power of Attorney	yes[4]	N/A	yes	no	yes[2]	no	yes	yes

[1] If the trust is revocable.

[2] If the written document specifically permits the trustee or attorney-in-fact to make such transfers.

[3] Can be created as a revocable or irrevocable trust.

[4] If it is a "springing" power of attorney.

BUYER BEWARE: NURSING HOME INSURANCE

BUYER BEWARE: NURSING HOME INSURANCE

Over the last decade, people have become increasingly aware of how quickly long-term care can wipe out their savings, and insurance companies have been just as quick to capitalize on that fear. "Nursing home insurance" has been advertised as protection against the costs of long-term nursing care. But for the most part, it provides overpriced, extremely limited benefits that cover only a small percentage of nursing facility costs.

A number of state insurance commissioners and consumer groups have studied this emerging type of coverage and have come to some very disturbing conclusions. Basically, they found the policies contained so many conditions and exclusions that *over 60% of people who bought nursing home insurance and later entered a nursing facility wound up collecting nothing at all.* And premiums paid by many others who bought insurance but never entered a nursing facility were wasted, too.

The studies also found that even when coverage did go into effect, the amounts paid were usually far below actual costs and lapsed before the nursing facility stay ended. More than half of all women over 65 and about a third of all men will enter a nursing facility at some point in their lives; half of those will stay more than six months and about 20% stay more than three years. Nursing facility insurance is supposed to be a hedge against the expensive possibility that long-term care will be needed. But these studies showed that despite all the promises and the money paid in nursing home insurance premiums, long-term care drained all the policyholders' personal savings, anyway.

The policies presently available are usually bad investments because, while they provide coverage for short-term, skilled nursing facility care following a hospital stay—often merely duplicating Medicare coverage—they do *not* provide coverage for long-term custodial care. And the few policies that do cover some long-term care

are expensive, difficult to qualify for and pay much less in benefits than actual nursing facility costs.

Yet it is long-term custodial care, of course, that Medicare does not cover and that most often drains the resident's and family's assets. Consumer activists are beginning to bring attention to the scandal of nursing home insurance, though, and perhaps consumer pressure will force insurance companies to offer better policies as public awareness grows.

A. SHOPPING FOR A POLICY

There are a few policies on the market that provide decent long-term coverage, but they are expensive.[1] And even if you qualify for such a policy, depending on your financial position, your money might be better invested elsewhere. (See Section H, Is Nursing Home Insurance Worth It?) Unfortunately, most policies provide lousy coverage, often at very high premiums. So, if you are interested in nursing home insurance, you must be a very careful consumer, and comparison shop thoroughly.

1. SOME WARNINGS ABOUT NURSING HOME INSURANCE

It is a mind-boggling task to find any kind of adequate insurance, but those searching for nursing home insurance should be forearmed with the following special forewarnings.

BEWARE OF PRETTY NUMBERS

Don't be blinded by the first numbers an insurance advertisement or agent shows you. Very often a company will show you low premiums and what seems like high benefits as if those were the only questions you needed to have answered. But if you pay the premiums but never see the benefits, you'll know too late that there are other important

---

[1]See Section G of this chapter, which lists several insurance companies offering policies with relatively comprehensive coverage.

questions to ask before buying the policy. This chapter discusses what those questions are, and the best answers to them.

BEWARE OF BROCHURES AND AGENTS

Insurance brochures and advertisements are often misleading and contradictory and are always incomplete. Brochures are intended to get you interested in insurance policies and to convince you how good they are—not to explain their pitfalls and problems or even to explain accurately how they work. And brochures do not bind an insurance company, so you cannot rely on their promises.

Insurance agents and brokers,[2] too, are in the business of selling policies, not of warning you why you should not buy one. Although agents are usually conscientious about not trying to sell a policy they know is not right for a customer, nursing home insurance is a new field, and most agents simply do not have much experience with it.

BEWARE OF MAIL-ORDER AND "LIMITED TIME" POLICIES

You have probably seen these advertising phrases before—they often come unsolicited in the mail: Limited Offer!; Once-in-a-Lifetime!; Never Before!; When this offer expires, you'll never get another chance!; One Month Only!

These one-time-only offers are usually misleading nonsense. The best advice may simply be to avoid any advertisement that uses an exclamation point. If it is a reputable insurance company with a legitimate policy to offer, the same or similar terms will be available to you at any time, except for premium increases because of a change in your age. So, no matter what the advertising says, don't be rushed into buying anything.

---

[2]In general, insurance agents represent one company or group of companies only. An agent speaks for the company and the company can be held responsible for most things an agent promises or claims about a policy. A broker, on the other hand, works independently and can offer policies from a number of different companies. A broker may be able to offer you more choices than an agent, but the broker's claims and promises about any policy are probably not binding against the insurance company.

■

CHECK THE COMPANY'S RELIABILITY

An independent insurance industry guide called *Best's Insurance Reports* rates individual insurance companies and policies. *Best's* gives a rating for a company's general reliability and financial status. You should consider only companies with a *Best's* rating of A+ or A. If you cannot get a *Best's* report at the library, the insurance agent or broker you deal with concerning the nursing home policy, or any other insurance agent or broker, should be able to get you a written statement of the company's *Best's* rating.

2. EXAMINE THE POLICY

When you are seriously considering a particular nursing home insurance policy, don't be content to just look at the policy in the insurance agent's office. Take home the complete policy—not a summary. After reading the policy carefully, ask the agent whatever questions you have about coverage and request explanations *in writing on behalf of the company*. These written clarifications must come either from an authorized company agent or other company representative, not from an independent broker. Ask for some evidence that the person giving you the explanation is authorized to speak on behalf of the company. If you do choose to purchase a policy after you have been given an extra written explanation, ask that the written explanation be attached to and made a part of your policy.

Some companies will not let you see the complete policy until you sign up to purchase it, but will give you a 30-day trial period during which you can return it and get your money back if you are not satisfied with its terms. Be suspicious of any company that will not show you its policy ahead of time. If you are tempted by the 30-day "free look," get the refund promise in writing. If there is no written guarantee that you can get your money back, forget about doing business with that insurance company.

3. MINIMUM STANDARDS

Because people's needs and financial situations vary, you must make up your own mind about what coverage you need and at what price. But *any* nursing home policy should contain certain terms. The checklist below sets out the minimum standards you should demand and refers you to the section in this chapter that discusses each standard in detail. After you have read this chapter all the way through, look back at the guide as you compare policies. Remember, don't jump at the first attractive numbers you see. If you do, you may pay the piper for years to come and get nothing in return.

■
_____

NURSING HOME INSURANCE MINIMUM STANDARDS GUIDE

If, after all things are considered, you decide to buy nursing home insurance, make sure that any policy you consider meets *at least* the following minimum standards:

1. The issuing company has a *Best's* rating of A+ or A. (See Section A1);
2. The policy has no requirement for a prior hospital or skilled nursing facility stay. (See Sections B1-B2);
3. It covers intermediate and custodial care in *any* level facility. (See Section B3);
4. It includes a written guarantee of Alzheimer's coverage, with details of how the company accepts Alzheimer's diagnosis. (See Sections B1, B6 and B7);
5. It guarantees a yearly adjustment of benefits for inflation. (See Section C);
6. It includes a deductible period of no more than 120 days, although 60 days is preferable. (See Section C4); and
7. The policy is "guaranteed renewable." (See Section D2).

B. CONDITIONS AND EXCLUSIONS

The biggest holes in nursing home policies are the many conditions and exclusions that apply to coverage. Insurance companies that promise high benefits at low premiums often do so because they so rarely have to pay off. So few of their policyholders meet all the conditions and exclusions that the policies are virtually worthless for coverage of long-term care. Whenever you consider a policy, look carefully at any conditions and exclusions, and particularly at the most common, ruinous ones listed below.

1. PRIOR HOSPITAL STAY

By some estimates, three-fourths of all nursing home insurance policies require a hospital stay of at least three days, within 7 to 30 days prior to entering a nursing facility, to qualify for any coverage. And while many nursing facility admissions do come from the hospital, only a very small number of long-term residents do. In other words, the requirement of a prior hospital stay eliminates coverage for the very kind of care one most hopes to be covered: long-term care because of chronic illness, frailty, or physical or mental impairment, including Alzheimer's disease.

Some people who purchased these policies and later discovered the prior hospitalization rule have actually wound up pleading with doctors and hospitals—or having to exaggerate their conditions—to spend the required three days in the hospital. So, to avoid the sorry situations of being needlessly hospitalized or having a worthless policy, do not buy any policy that requires a prior hospital stay.

2. PRIOR SKILLED NURSING FACILITY STAY

A number of policies require that before they will pay for residence in an intermediate or personal care facility, you must have spent up to two weeks in a skilled nursing facility within a certain time period before admission to the long-term care facility. And many policies also require that the time spent in a skilled nursing facility must be primarily for skilled nursing care, eliminating people not admitted by a doctor for daily skilled nursing care. Again, this condition tends to exclude people with chronic illnesses or impairments. This type of policy may cover only people who enter a facility after an acute episode of illness, injury or surgery.

Some insurance companies are so devious that they actually require not only a prior skilled nursing facility stay, but also that *their* policy have covered that stay before they will pay for any other care. In other words, if Medicare covered your costs in a skilled nursing facility, the insurance policy does not pick up when Medicare leaves off—the reason you bought the policy in the first place.

■
_____

REPEAT WARNING

Do not buy any policy with a requirement of a prior skilled nursing facility stay.

3. COVERAGE IN SKILLED NURSING FACILITIES ONLY

Some policies, with or without a prior hospitalization requirement, will provide coverage only for care given *in* a Medicare-certified skilled nursing facility. But long-term chronic care is not available in many of these facilities, and short-term skilled care is well covered by Medicare. Again, the insurance policy fails to cover precisely the long-term care costs one hopes to protect against.

Even if one of these policies does not require you to receive regular skilled nursing care and does pay for intermediate care, you must find a skilled nursing facility that will admit you as a long-term, intermediate or custodial resident. And even if you find one, the daily rate will be much higher than in an intermediate or personal care facility. Since private insurance policies pay only a portion of daily costs, you would wind up paying much more than you should just to get the insurance company to pay anything. Such coverage is a bad bet.

4. SAME ILLNESS OR CONDITION

Some policies that require prior hospitalization or a stay in a skilled nursing facility also require that admission to a long-term care facility be for the same illness or condition. Your doctor must submit a written statement of the reason for your admission to long-term care, and it must match the diagnosis that led to your admission.

This may not seem like a problem, but suppose, for example, a disabling condition or frailty causes a fall that results in injuries requiring hospitalization. Once the injuries are treated, it would be the original condition or frailty that might require long-term care, not the injuries that caused the hospitalization. And that would disqualify the policyholder from coverage.

5. PRE-EXISTING CONDITION EXCLUSION

Like most other health insurance policies, nursing home insurance almost always excludes coverage for residential care occasioned by an illness or condition which has been diagnosed or treated within a certain time before the starting date of the policy. The time period before the policy goes into effect can be anywhere from six months to two years. If you are purchasing a nursing home policy after you have been actively treated for a medical condition which you believe might lead to residential care, you must pay particular attention to the pre-existing exclusion clauses.

The exclusions work in several ways. Some policies exclude coverage for a certain period of time after you have become a resident because of the pre-existing condition. For the first three months, six months or a year, you will be personally responsible for nursing home costs and then the insurance coverage will kick in.

■
_____

WARNING

Some nursing home policies permanently exclude coverage if, during the exclusion period, you enter a nursing facility as a result of a pre-existing condition. Avoid such policies no matter what else they might offer. The effect of this exclusion is that you would never receive any benefits from the insurance company no matter how long you remained a nursing facility resident. (See the discussion, below.)

Look instead for the shortest pre-residence period and the shortest exclusion period.

6. PERMANENT EXCLUSIONS

These are the capital punishment clauses of insurance policies. Insurance companies will sell you a policy and collect premiums for years, even though there was little hope from the beginning that you could collect the benefits because you have been treated within the pre-existing condition period for an excluded condition. These policies will never pay if you fit into any of these categories. Check carefully for permanent exclusion clauses.

MEDICAL CONDITION (TOTAL EXCLUSION)

Some policies exclude from coverage anyone previously diagnosed or treated for certain conditions, whether or not they have anything to do with admission to a residential care facility. The conditions usually include mental illness, alcohol or chemical dependency, certain heart diseases, certain cancers, diabetes and Alzheimer's disease. (See the special warning on Alzheimer's in Section B7.)

With many of these conditions you would know in advance whether or not you would be excluded. But some may remain hidden. What if, for example, you had once been taking too much sleeping medication and your doctor changed or stopped the medication? Does that amount to "chemical dependency?" If possible, you and your doctor should examine your medical history carefully and compare it with a policy's permanent exclusions before you sign up for the insurance.

MEDICAL CONDITION (ADMISSION)

Some policies exclude the same kinds of conditions as mentioned just above, but only if your admission to residential care was for treatment of, or resulted from, the excluded condition. This is not as severe a restriction, but it still makes the policy a gamble. If you have had an excluded condition, you probably won't know whether it will be what leads to nursing facility residence. If you are being actively treated for an excluded condition, or are having personal care difficulties because of one, check carefully whether a medical condition exclusion would disqualify you from coverage.

AGE

All insurance companies charge higher premiums to older nursing home policy buyers. But some companies will not even sell a policy to someone over a certain age: 70, 75 or 80. If this sounds to you like age discrimination, you're right, it is. If it sounds illegal, it's not. It's called "free enterprise."

PRIOR NURSING FACILITY RESIDENCE

A number of policies are not available to anyone who has previously been a resident in a nursing facility for a certain length of time. Usually these exclusions permit a brief prior stay—while recovering from an acute illness, for example. No policies are available to current residents of a nursing facility.

7. SPECIAL WARNING ON ALZHEIMER'S EXCLUSIONS

Alzheimer's disease is one of the leading causes of the need for long-term residential care. But while the memory loss, disorientation and loss of motor coordination associated with Alzheimer's reduces a person's ability to handle personal care without assistance, Alzheimer's sufferers frequently live for many years without requiring skilled medical care. They would greatly benefit from insurance coverage for long-term custodial care.

But the way many nursing home policies work, Alzheimer's residents are often left without coverage even if nothing in the policy specifically excludes Alzheimer's and often even if the policy claims it does cover Alzheimer's admissions.

A review of common policy exclusions shows how this trap works:

PRIOR HOSPITALIZATION OR SKILLED NURSING FACILITY STAY

Since most Alzheimer's sufferers do not require acute medical care before needing long-term personal care, a policy that requires a prior hospital or skilled nursing facility stay would exclude most Alzheimer's residents.

MENTAL OR NERVOUS DISORDER EXCLUSION

Many policies exclude coverage if admission to a facility is occasioned by a "mental or nervous disorder." And although Alzheimer's is an illness with an organic cause, it is difficult to diagnose precisely. Since its symptoms often resemble forms of mental or emotional illness, the resident's family may be required to prove to the insurance company that the resident's problem really is an organic disease. As you might imagine, many people have lost this battle with insurance companies.

PRE-EXISTING CONDITION EXCLUSION

As discussed above, many policies exclude coverage if admission to residential care results from a condition for which the resident was diagnosed or treated within a certain period before the policy went into effect. The extra catch with Alzheimer's is that because it is difficult to diagnose, sometimes a person is treated within the exclusion period for a problem only later understood to be related to Alzheimer's. In such a case, the insurance company might claim the pre-existing condition exclusion. It is another good reason not to buy a policy with a permanent pre-existing condition exclusion. If it is only a temporary exclusion, at least there will be some coverage for a long-term residence.

The best way to make sure of adequate coverage for Alzheimer's is to have a policy with no requirement of prior hospital or skilled nursing facility stay. The policy should state clearly that it covers admissions to residential facilities due to Alzheimer's and that the company accepts the written diagnosis of a physician as proof that a patient has Alzheimer's rather than a mental or nervous disorder, if such disorders are excluded from coverage.

C. BENEFITS PAID

1. SET DAILY AMOUNT

Unlike most health insurance, almost all nursing home policies pay a fixed daily amount regardless of the cost of care. And that amount is usually well below actual cost. Benefits vary from $10 to $100 per day, depending on premiums charged and conditions imposed on coverage. Since residential care facilities currently cost anywhere from $30 to $200 per day (see the discussion of Inflation Adjustment, below), you can see what a gaping hole these policies often leave, assuming they pay any benefits at all.

Look for a policy that pays $75 to $100 per day—for custodial care, not skilled care. But consider it a good buy only if the premium is competitive and there is an inflation adjustment on the benefit amount.

2. INFLATION ADJUSTMENT

A benefit of $80 per day seems reasonable given today's average daily nursing facility costs, but you are probably not buying a policy to protect against today's costs. You might not enter a facility for five, ten or twenty years. Estimates are that nursing facility costs will double in only ten years, and those are conservative estimates which assume that costs will only increase as fast as inflation.

At that rate, an intermediate care facility that today costs $80 per day may cost $160 per day in ten years. If you buy a policy now that pays an $80 per day benefit, you would still have to pay $80 per day out of your pocket. If your stay in the facility is two years—an average length—you would have to pay over $56,000 above what the insurance pays. If that amount will eat up your savings anyway, the years you spent paying insurance premiums to protect those savings will have been fruitless.

One way to help protect against inevitable increases in nursing facility costs is to find a policy with a built-in inflation adjustment clause. The standard is an increase in benefits of five per cent per year. Some policies link benefits to rises in the cost of living, but even that does not fully protect you since nursing facility costs have consistently risen faster than inflation. They are, however, usually the best inflation adjustments you can get with a nursing facility policy.

One further point: Almost all insurance companies charge extra for inflation protection.

3. BENEFITS VARY WITH LEVEL OF CARE

Read a policy carefully to see if, and by how much, benefit amounts vary with the level of care you receive. Policies are often advertised by the benefit amount paid for skilled nursing facility care, with lower payments for intermediate or custodial care buried in the fine print. But the benefit for skilled nursing care is, in fact, the least important. Skilled nursing care tends to be relatively short-term, and Medicare pays for much of it.

The most important figure is the custodial care benefit—the amount paid for daily care that does not involve skilled medical care, but which includes room, board and personal assistance with routine daily activities such as eating and bathing. Since it is custodial care that often continues for months and years, and that is not covered by Medicare, the insurance policy's custodial care benefits are the most important. And the custodial care amount is often only half of the advertised skilled nursing benefit.

4. DEDUCTIBLE (ELIMINATION) PERIODS

Almost all policies have a deductible period at the beginning of the nursing facility stay during which they pay nothing. A few have a deductible amount of money, instead of number of days, which you must pay before the insurance coverage begins. Deductible periods vary from 10 days up to 100 days after admission. And premiums vary with the length of the deductible: the shorter the deductible, the higher the premium.

Since the cost of long-term custodial care is probably what you are most concerned about protecting against, then a long deductible period may not be such a bad thing if it means significant monthly premium savings. This is particularly true if you are buying your policy when you are only in your 50s or 60s and will probably be paying the premium for a long time.

■
_____

WARNING

A few policies that require a skilled nursing facility stay before they will cover custodial care are worded so that they won't cover custodial care unless the insurance company has first actually *paid* for skilled nursing facility care. But if your stay in a skilled nursing facility is shorter—usually less than 30 days—than your deductible period, the insurance will have paid nothing for that care and thus *will not pay for any custodial care, either*.

5. MAXIMUM PAYMENTS

Most policies have a limit on the total amount of money they will pay under the policy. A few policies specify a dollar limit, but most use total number of days or months of coverage or a combination of the two. Half of all nursing facility stays are for over six months, but 80% are for under three years. Therefore, a three to four-year benefit period is probably sufficient, with five to six years advisable if the cost is not significantly greater. Two years is the minimum you should accept.

Some policies have different maximums for different levels of care. The insurance company may flash a reassuringly large amount as the limit of the policy benefits, but closer inquiry may reveal a much smaller limit on long-term custodial care. Make sure you see the fine print that explains the maximum payments for all levels of care.

D. PREMIUMS

1. INITIAL PREMIUMS

The cost of initial premiums varies with your age as well as with the quality and amounts of coverage. Insurance companies offer monthly premiums for nursing home coverage to people in the youngest age groups (55 to 59) which often run between $25 and $40 per month. The lowest premiums, however, provide the smallest benefits with the greatest exclusions, conditions and limitations. If you are age 75, for example, and want broad coverage with high benefits, you will have to pay $300 to $400 per month.

But as you have already seen, premium cost and benefit amounts are not the only factors to consider. You must take into account conditions and exclusions, levels of care, deductibles and maximum total payments. And with regard to premiums, you must also consider whether the insurance company can *raise* the premiums after you've bought the policy.

2. RENEWABILITY

An insurance company that issues you a nursing facility policy today may no longer be issuing such policies ten years from now. Or it may not even be in business. If the company wants to get out of the nursing facility insurance business, can it cancel your policy? If its profits are slipping, can it raise your premium rates? Can it transfer your policy to another company where your premiums will be much higher because by now you are in an older age group?

These questions should be specifically covered in your policy under the heading, "renewability." For your protection, you should only buy a policy that is "noncancelable" or "guaranteed renewable," as explained below. Do not buy a policy that is "conditionally renewable" or "optionally renewable."

3. WAIVER OF PREMIUMS

Make sure there is a provision that once you have been in a covered facility for a certain period of time (usually 90 to 120 days), further payment of premiums is waived. In other words, look for a provision that once the insurance company starts paying you, you stop paying them. Otherwise, the premiums will eat up all your benefits. Charges for these provisions may vary.

■

INSURANCE WORDS TO THE WISE

A few definitions may help you through the morass of words
that make up insurance policies.

Noncancelable: A noncancelable policy is one that
cannot be canceled by the company or any successor
company—unless you don't pay your premiums. And premiums
cannot be raised during the life of the policy except as
specifically spelled out in the original policy. There may be a
built-in rise in premiums, for example, to account for inflation.

Guaranteed renewable: The policy cannot be
canceled by the insurer or its successor company, but the insurer
can raise premiums for a whole group or class of policyholders,
such as a particular age group. Competition for customers
supposedly limits the willingness of companies to raise
premiums for an entire group nationwide. This is not as good a
guarantee as with a noncancelable policy, but it is more
common and is acceptable if the other terms and conditions of
the policy are favorable.

Conditionally renewable: With these policies, the
insurer can refuse to renew the policy at the end of its stated
term, or it can raise premiums as much as it likes for a group or
class of policyholders, or within a geographic area. It still cannot
do so individually or on the basis of particular levels of health,
but this kind of policy gives the insurer too much control. It
allows a company to get out of policies if rates and benefits later
prove to be less profitable than estimated, placing all the
business risk on the policyholder's shoulders. A conditionally
renewable policy is a bad risk.

Optionally renewable: Unfortunately, with these
policies, all the options are held by the insurance companies.
The company can refuse to renew the policy or can raise
premiums almost at will, such as when you reach a new age
group, or when the monthly profit statement starts to sag. Never
buy a policy that is renewable at the insurance company's
option.

E. HOME HEALTH CARE COVERAGE UNDER NURSING HOME POLICIES

Some nursing home insurance policies provide for limited home health care coverage. Because the coverage is limited, do not buy nursing home insurance for home care coverage alone. However, if you are considering buying a policy for residential long-term care protection, try to find one that also offers home care coverage.

Nursing facility policies usually cover only a limited number of home health care visits, with conditions similar to or even more restrictive than Medicare. Benefits are usually only a small portion of what Medicare does not pay—and take effect only after both the policy's and Medicare's deductible are reached. The maximum daily benefit these policies pay is usually only half their daily nursing facility benefit.

Nonetheless, if all other things seem equal between competing nursing facility policies, substantial home care coverage is something to consider.

F. WHERE TO LOOK FOR NURSING FACILITY INSURANCE

The only way to find a nursing home insurance policy with the highest benefits and widest coverage for the lowest premium price is to comparison shop, then shop some more. A good independent insurance broker may help you get started finding and comparing policies, but do not depend on a single agent for all your information. In general, insurance brokers know little about nursing home policies, and are often limited to the few companies with which they regularly do business. Try to find a broker who handles more than one kind of nursing facility policy and who has some experience in this relatively new field. When you ask a broker to locate policies for you, insist that all policies must at least meet the Minimum Standards Guide listed in Section 1 of this chapter.

If you have trouble locating policies to compare, get the names and addresses of companies that sell nursing home policies through your state Department of Insurance, through your state or Area Agency on Aging, at your local library, or from the Health Insurance

Association of America, Consumer Information Service, 1001
Pennsylvania Avenue, NW, Washington, DC 20004-2599.

G. SOME ACCEPTABLE POLICIES

Because the terms, conditions, premiums and benefit amounts of
insurance policies change so frequently, the provisions of specific
policies are not listed here. By the time you read this, any policy
discussed may no longer exist or may have changed significantly. Also,
because the advisability of purchasing any policy depends on your
personal financial situation, no recommendations are made here about
any particular policy.

However, to help you and your broker begin comparison
shopping, several insurance policies are listed below that currently
meet the minimum requirements outlined in the Minimum Standards
Guide listed earlier in this chapter. This does not guarantee these
policies still meet the minimum standards, or that they are a wise
purchase for you. A thorough examination of your financial situation
and of the terms of these and other policies is the only way you can
make that decision.[3]

- Aetna Life & Casualty, Long-Term Care Plan B
- AIG Life, Nursing Home Insurance
- AMEX Life, Long-Term Care Plan
- CNA, Convalescent Care Plan, High Option
- John Hancock, Protect Care (Comprehensive)
- Mutual of Omaha, Long-Term Care Plus
- New York Life, Group Long-Term Care
- North American Life & Casualty Co., Assured Care Plus, Plan B
- Travelers, Independent Care

---

[3] *Consumer Reports*, a consumer information magazine, did a comprehensive study of
many long-term care insurance policies in its May, 1988 issue and updated the
information in October, 1989. These articles, plus any further updates, could be a
valuable reference when you begin to look for a policy. *Consumer Reports* can be
found at any local library.

H. IS NURSING HOME INSURANCE WORTH IT?

The only way you can determine whether nursing home insurance is a good value for you is to gauge how much you would pay in premiums before entering a facility, based on your age and general health, and measure that amount against both the benefits you would receive and the remaining unpaid costs. Since what you are protecting against is the cost of long-term care, make your calculations based on estimates of two-year and three-year facility residence. Consider, too, the possibility that you will never be in a nursing facility at all, or will be in one for such a short time that the policy will not pay any benefits.

You can see that after determining which policies have acceptable conditions, exclusions and deductible periods, deciding whether a policy is worthwhile becomes primarily a math problem. If you do not have much disposable income to spend on premiums and do not have a lot of savings to protect against nursing facility costs, a nursing facility insurance policy is probably a bad idea.

Example: If you had $10,000 in savings and had spent another $300 per month for 10 years for a nursing home policy that paid $50 per day, a nursing facility that cost $80 per day would run through those savings and force you to rely on Medicaid after only 11 months. If you had not spent the money on the insurance policy, however, you might have been forced to rely on Medicaid somewhat sooner than 11 months, but for 10 years you would have had the use of the $36,000, plus interest, you paid in premiums.

■
_____

LIFE INSURANCE COVERAGE OF LONG-TERM CARE

About two dozen insurance companies have provisions in their life insurance policies that permit a policyholder to pay an increased premium of approximately five per cent to receive nursing home coverage. The monthly benefits paid by this coverage are usually about two per cent of what the death benefit would have been. Collecting on the nursing home coverage, however, would reduce or eliminate payment of the death benefit.

Although it is not financially advisable to purchase life insurance just for nursing home coverage, if you already have life insurance, it is worth checking with your insurance representative to see if such nursing home coverage is available under your policy.

In general, if in addition to your home you have substantial assets and income—over $100,000 in assets and over $20,000 per year in income—then a good nursing home insurance policy with high benefits might be a reasonable investment. However, even if you do have sizable assets, a business adviser may show you that an annuity, certificates of deposit, investment in your home or other investment of the same money you would pay an insurance company makes more sense for you. Whatever your situation, it is probably a good idea to consult with someone knowledgeable in long-term financial planning about the wisdom of investing in a nursing home policy. Do not base your decision solely on advice from an insurance agent or broker who is trying to sell you a nursing home policy.

appendix

RESOURCE DIRECTORY

AGING, STATE OFFICES

These are the central offices in each state, run by the state government, which provide general information and referrals to all the specific agencies within the state which provide services for elders.

ALABAMA
Commission on Aging
136 Catoma Street
Montgomery, AL 36130
(205) 261-5743

ALASKA
Older Alaskans Commission
Department of Administration
Pouch C
Juneau, AK 99811-0209
(907) 465-3250

ARIZONA
Aging & Adult Administration
Department of Economic
Security
1400 West Washington Street
Phoenix, AZ 85007
(602) 542-4446

ARKANSAS
Division of Aging, Adult Services
Department of Social
Rehabilitative Services
Donaghey Building
Suite 1417
7th and Main Streets
Little Rock, AR 72201
(501) 682-8500

CALIFORNIA
Department on Aging
1600 K Street
Sacramento, CA 95814
(916) 322-5290

COLORADO
Aging and Adult Services
Division
2200 West Alameda Street
Denver, CO 80223
(303) 936-3666

CONNECTICUT
Department on Aging
175 Main Street
Hartford, CT 06106
(203) 566-3238

DELAWARE
Division on Aging
Department of Health and Social
Services
1901 North Dupont Highway
New Castle, DE 19720
(302) 421-6791

**DISTRICT OF
COLUMBIA**
Office on Aging
1424 K Street, NW
2nd Floor
Washington, DC 20005
(202) 724-5625

FLORIDA
Program Office of Aging and
Services
Department of Health and
Rehabilitation Services
1317 Winewood Boulevard
Tallahassee, FL 32399-0700
(904) 488-8922

GEORGIA
Office of Aging
Room 632
878 Peachtree Street, NE
Atlanta, GA 30309
(404) 894-5333

GUAM
Public Health & Social Services
Government of Guam
Agana, Guam 96910

HAWAII
Executive Office on Aging
Office of the Governor
Room 241
335 Merchant Street
Honolulu, HI 96813
(808) 548-2593

IDAHO
Office on Aging
Room 108—Capitol Building
Boise, ID 83720
(208) 334-3833

ILLINOIS
Department on Aging
421 E. Capitol Avenue
Springfield, IL 62701
(217) 785-2870

INDIANA
Department of Aging and
Adult Community Services
251 North Illinois Street
P.O. Box 7083
Indianapolis, IN 46207-7083
(317) 232-7006

IOWA
Department of Elder Affairs
Suite 236, Jewett Building
914 Grand Avenue
Des Moines, IA 50309
(515) 281-5187

KANSAS
Department on Aging
Docking State Office Building
Rm 122-S
915 SW Harrison Street
Topeka, KS 66612-1500
(913) 296-4986

KENTUCKY
Division for Aging Services
Department of Human
Resources
CHR Building—6th Floor
275 East Main Street
Frankfort, KY 40621
(502) 564-6930

LOUISIANA
Office of Elderly Affairs
P.O. Box 80374
Baton Rouge, LA 70898-0374
(504) 925-1700

MAINE
Bureau of Maine's Elderly
Department of Human Services
State House—Station #11
1 Amherst Street
Augusta, ME 04333
(207) 289-2561

MARYLAND
Office on Aging
State Office Building
301 West Preston Street, Room
1004
Baltimore, MD 21201
(301) 225-1100

MASSACHUSETTS
Executive Office of Elder Affairs
38 Chauncy Street
Boston, MA 02111
(617) 727-7750

MICHIGAN
Office of Services to the Aging
P.O. Box 30029
Lansing, MI 48909
(517) 373-8230

MINNESOTA
Board on Aging
444 Lafayette Road
St. Paul, MN 55155-3843
(612) 296-2544

MISSISSIPPI
Council on Aging
421 West Pascagoula Street
Jackson, MS 39203
(601) 949-2070

MISSOURI
Division on Aging
Department of Social Services
P.O. Box 1337
2701 West Main Street
Jefferson City, MO 65102
(314) 751-3082

MONTANA
Community Services Division
P.O. Box 4210
Helena, MT 59604
(no phone listing)

NEBRASKA
Department on Aging
301 Centennial Mall—South
P.O. Box 95044
Lincoln, NE 68509
(402) 471-2306

NEVADA
Division on Aging
Department of Human
Resources
505 East King Street, Room 101
Carson City, NV 89710
(702) 885-4210

NEW HAMPSHIRE
Council on Aging
6 Hazen Drive
Concord, NH 03301
(603) 271-4680

NEW JERSEY
Division on Aging
Department of Community
Affairs
101 South Broad Street
CN807
Trenton, NJ 08625-0807
(609) 292-4833

NEW MEXICO
State Agency on Aging
224 East Palace Avenue, 4th
Floor
La Villa Rivera Building
Santa Fe, NM 87501
(505) 827-7640

NEW YORK
Office for the Aging
Empire State Plaza
Agency Building #2
Albany, NY 12223
(518) 474-4425

NORTH CAROLINA
Division on Aging
1985 Umpstead Drive
Raleigh, NC 27603
(919) 733-3983

NORTH DAKOTA
Aging Services
State Capitol Building
600 East Boulevard Avenue
Bismarck, ND 58505-0250
(701) 224-2577

OHIO
Department on Aging
50 West Broad Street, 9th Floor
Columbus, OH 43215
(614) 466-5500

OKLAHOMA
Special Unit on Aging
Department of Human Services
P.O. Box 25352
Oklahoma City, OK 73125
(405) 521-2281

OREGON
Senior Services Division
313 Public Service Building
Salem, OR 97310
(503) 378-4728

PENNSYLVANIA
Department on Aging
231 State Street
Harrisburg, PA 17101-1195
(717) 783-1550

PUERTO RICO
Gericulture Commission
Department of Social Services
P.O. Box 11398
Santurce, PR 00910
(809) 721-3141 or 722-0225

RHODE ISLAND
Department of Elderly Affairs
160 Pine Street
Providence, RI 02903
(401) 277-2858

(AMERICAN) SAMOA
Territorial Administration on
Aging
Office of the Governor
Pago Pago, American Samoa
96779-9011
(684) 633-1252

SOUTH CAROLINA
Commission on Aging
400 Arbor Lake Drive
Columbia, SC 29223
(803) 735-0210

SOUTH DAKOTA
Office of Adult Services
700 Governors Drive
Pierre, SD 57501-2291
(605) 773-3656

TENNESSEE
Commission on Aging
706 Church Street, Suite 201
Nashville, TN 37219-5573
(615) 741-2056

TEXAS
Department on Aging
P.O. Box 12786 Capitol Station
Austin, TX 78711
(512) 444-2727

UTAH
Division of Aging & Adult
Services
Department of Social Services
120 North 200 West, Room 401
Salt Lake City, UT 84103
(801) 538-3910

VERMONT
Office on Aging
103 South Main Street
Waterbury, VT 05676
(802) 241-2400

VIRGINIA
Department on Aging
700 East Franklin Street, 10th
Floor
Richmond, VA 23219
(804) 225-2271

VIRGIN ISLANDS
Commission on Aging
6F Havensight Mall
St. Thomas, VI 00801
(809) 774-5884

WASHINGTON
Aging & Adult Services
Administration
Department of Social & Health
Services
Mail Stop OB-44A
Olympia, WA 98504
(206) 586-3768

WEST VIRGINIA
Commission on Aging
Holly Grove—State Capitol
Charleston, WV 25305
(304) 348-3317

WISCONSIN
Commission on Aging
217 S. Hamilton, Suite 300
Madison, WI 53703
(608) 266-2536

WYOMING
Commission on Aging
139 Hathaway Building
Cheyenne, WY 82002
(307) 777-7986

CAREGIVER SUPPORT GROUPS

Children of Aging Parents
2761 Trenton Road
Levittown, PA 19056
(215) 945-6900

Children of Aging Parents is a nonprofit organization that provides support and information to the families and friends of the dependent elderly. It maintains a directory of self-help support groups for family caregivers, publishes a number of helpful pamphlets for caregivers and puts out a newsletter that provides up-to-date information on programs for the elderly and their families. Enclose $1 and a self-addressed, stamped envelope with any request for information.

HOME CARE

NATIONAL ORGANIZATIONS

These organizations all provide information and referrals both to specific home care providers in your area and also to state and local home care organizations, which can in turn provide you with even more detailed information and referrals. Following this list of national organizations is a list of state home care associations.

Joint Commission for
Accreditation of Health
Care Organizations
875 North Michigan Avenue
Chicago IL 60611
(302) 642-6061

National Association for Home Care
519 C Street, NE
Washington, DC 20002
(202) 547-7424

Family Service Association
of America
National Office
11700 West Lake Park Drive
Milwaukee, WI 53224

Aging Network Services
Topaz House
4400 East-West Highway, Suite 907
Bethesda, MD 20814
(301) 657-4329

Visiting Nurse Associations
and Services
1129 Macklind Avenue
St. Louis, MO 63110
(314) 533-9680

American Hospital Association
Division of Ambulatory Care
840 North Lake Shore Drive
Chicago, IL 60611
(312) 280-6216

National Association of
Meal Programs
Box 6344
604 West North Avenue
Pittsburgh, PA 15212
(no phone listing)

National Council on the Aging
600 Maryland Avenue SW, West
Wing 100
Washington, DC 20024
(202) 479-1200

STATE ASSOCIATIONS

If your state is not listed here, you can obtain information on the association in your state by contacting the National Association for Home Care, 519 C Street, NE, Washington, DC 20002; (202) 547-7424.

ARIZONA
Arizona Association for Home
Care
20 East Main Street, Suite 710
Mesa, AZ 85201
(602) 969-0399

ARKANSAS
Arkansas Association for
Home Health Agencies
1501 North University, Suite 400
Little Rock, AR 72207
(501) 224-7878

CALIFORNIA
California Association for
Health Services at Home
660 J. Street, Suite 290
Sacramento, CA 95814
(916) 443-8055

COLORADO
Colorado Association of Home
Health Agencies
7600 East Arapahoe Road, Suite
316
Englewood, CO 80112
(303) 694-4728

CONNECTICUT
Connecticut Association
for Home Care
110 Barnes Rd.
P.O. Box 90
Wallingford, CT 06492
(203) 265-8931

**DISTRICT OF
COLUMBIA**
Capitol Home Health
Association
519 C. Street, NE
Washington, D.C. 20002
(202) 547-7424

GEORGIA
Georgia Association of Home
Health Agencies
1260 South Omni International
Atlanta, GA 30303
(404) 984-9704

ILLINOIS
Illinois Home Care Council
2008 Dempster Street
Evanston, IL 60202
(312) 328-6654

INDIANA
Indiana Association of Home
Health Agencies
8888 Keystone Crossing, Suite
1000
Indianapolis, IN 46240
(317) 844-6630

KENTUCKY
Kentucky Home Health
Association
153 Patchen Drive, Suite 40
Lexington, KY 40517
(606) 268-2574

MASSACHUSETTS
Massachusetts Association of
Community Health Agencies
100 Boylston Street, Suite 724
Boston, MA 02116
(617) 482-8830

MISSISSIPPI
Mississippi Home Health
Association
812 North President Street
Jackson, MS 39202
(601) 948-6442

MISSOURI
Missouri Association of Home
Health Agencies
1125 Madison Street
Jefferson City, MO 65101
(314) 635-4663

NEW JERSEY
Home Health Agency Assembly
of New Jersey
760 Alexander Road, CN-1
Princeton, NJ 08540
(609) 452-8855

NEW YORK
Home Care Associations of
New York State
1 Columbia Place
Albany, NY 12207
(518) 426-8764

NORTH CAROLINA
North Carolina Association
for Home Care
1005 Dresser Court
Raleigh, NC 27609
(919) 878-0500

OHIO
Ohio Council of Home Health
Agencies
5008 Pine Creek Drive, Suite B
Westerville, OH 43081
(614) 898-7684

PENNSYLVANIA
Pennsylvania Association of
Home Health Agencies
1500 North 2nd Street, 3rd Floor
Harrisburg, PA 17102
(717) 233-3363

TENNESSEE
Tennessee Association for Home
Health
4711 Trousdale Drive
Nashville, TN 37220
(615) 331-0463

TEXAS
Texas Association of Home
Health Agencies
1016 La Posada Drive, Suite 129
Austin, TX 78752
(512) 459-4303

VERMONT
Vermont Assembly of Home
Health Agencies
52 State Street
Montpelier, VT 05602
(802) 229-0579

WASHINGTON
Home Care Association of
Washington
P.O. Box C-2016
Edmonds, WA 98020-0999
(206) 774-7479

WEST VIRGINIA
West Virginia Council of
Home Health Agencies
P.O. Box 4227
Star City, WV 26504-4227
(304) 363-5431

WISCONSIN
Wisconsin Homecare
Organization
(mailing)
P.O. Box 4288
Madison, WI 53711
(street)
6441 Enterprise Lane
Madison, WI 53719
(608) 274-8118

INSURANCE—NURSING FACILITY

The following are sources of information about nursing facility insurance policies available in your state.

HEALTH INSURANCE ASSOCIATION OF AMERICA
Consumer Information Service
1025 Connecticut Avenue, NW, Suite 1200
Washington, DC 20036
(202) 223-7780
hotline: 800-942-4242

STATE DEPARTMENTS OF INSURANCE
Each state has a government agency that regulates the sale of insurance. There should be a listing for an insurance department under the listings in the white pages of the telephone directory for Government Offices. It can provide you with a list of companies authorized to sell long-term insurance in your state.

STATE OFFICES ON AGING
Like the Departments of Insurance, the Office on Aging in your state should have a current list of long-term care policies authorized for sale in your state. The Offices on Aging are listed earlier in this Resource Directory.

LEGAL ASSISTANCE

The following groups either provide or give referrals for, protection of the legal rights of the elderly. Some provide information on government programs and legislation affecting the elderly.

National Senior Citizens Law Center
2025 M Street, NW, Suite 400
Washington, DC 20036
(202) 887-5280

Older Women's League
730 11th Street, NW, Suite 300
Washington, DC 20001
(202) 783-6686

National Council of Senior Citizens
925 15th Street, NW
Washington, DC 20005
(202) 624-9500

Gray Panthers
National Office
3635 Chestnut Street
Philadelphia, PA 19104

Legal Counsel for the Elderly
American Association of Retired Persons
1331 H Street, NW, Suite 10005
Washington, DC 20005
(202) 234-0970

LICENSING AND CERTIFICATION

AGENCIES ON NURSING CARE STANDARDS

These are the agencies in each state that establish standards to be met by home health care agencies, nursing facilities and individual health care providers such as independent home health care workers. They can provide you with information regarding whether any particular health care provider or facility is licensed or certified by the state and what state standards must be met for that license or certification.

See also the list of Nursing Facility License & Certification Offices immediately following this one.

ALABAMA
Bureau of Licensing &
Certification
Alabama Department of Public
Health
434 Monroe Street
Montgomery, AL 36130-1701
(205) 261-5113

ALASKA
Health Facilities Licensing &
Certification
Department of Health & Social
Services
4433 Business Park Boulevard
Building M
Anchorage AK 99503
(907) 561-2171

ARIZONA
Health Care Institutions &
Licensing
Department of Health Services
701 East Jefferson, Suite 300
Phoenix, AZ 85034
(602) 255-1177

ARKANSAS
Medicare Certification
Arkansas Department of Health
4815 West Markham Street, Slot 9
Little Rock, AR 72205-3867
(501) 661-2201

CALIFORNIA
Licensing & Certification of
Health Services
1800 3rd Street, Suite 200
Sacramento, CA 95814
(916) 445-2070

COLORADO
Health Facilities Regulation
Division
Department of Health
4210 East 11th Avenue
Denver, CO 80220
(303) 331-4930

CONNECTICUT
Licensing & Certification
Division
of Hospital & Medical Care
Department of Health Services
150 Washington Street
Hartford, CT 06106
(203) 566-1073

DELAWARE
Health Facilities Licensing &
Certification
Department of Health and Social
Services
3000 Newport Gap Pike
Wilmington, DE 19808
(302) 995-6674

**DISTRICT OF
COLUMBIA**
Service Facilities
Regulation Administration
Department of Consumer &
Regulatory Affairs
614 H Street, NW, Room 1014
Washington, DC 20001
(202) 727-7190

FLORIDA
Office of Licensure and
Certification
2727 Mahan Drive
Tallahassee, FL 32308
(904) 487-3513

GEORGIA
Laboratory Licensure &
Development Section
878 Peachtree Street, NE, Room
814
Atlanta, GA 30309
(404) 894-5841

HAWAII
Hospital & Medical Facilities
Branch
Department of Health
P.O. Box 3378
Honolulu, HI 96801
(808) 548-5935

IDAHO
Facilities Standards Program
Department of Health and Welfare
450 West State Street
Boise, ID 83720
(208) 334-6626

ILLINOIS
Bureau of Long-Term Care
Illinois Department of Public Health
525 West Jefferson, 5th Floor
Springfield, IL 62761
(217) 785-9184

INDIANA
Bureau of Health Institution
Standards
State Board of Health
1330 West Michigan Street,
Room 336
Indianapolis, IN 46206
(317) 633-8442

IOWA
Division of Health Facilities
Department of Inspections and
Appeals
Lucas State Office Building, 3rd
Floor
Des Moines, IA 50319
(515) 281-4294

KANSAS
Bureau of Adult & Child Care
Kansas Department of Health &
Environment
Landon State Office Building,
Suite 1001
900 SW Jackson Street
Topeka, KS 66612
(913) 296-1260

KENTUCKY
Division for Licensure &
Regulation
Cabinet for Human Resources
Building
275 East Main Street
Frankfort, KY 40621
(502) 564-2800

LOUISIANA
Division of Licensure &
Certification
Department of Health & Human
Resources
P.O. Box 3767
Baton Rouge, LA 70821
(504) 342-5774

MAINE
Division of Licensure &
Certification
249 Western Avenue
Augusta, ME 04333
(207) 289-2606

MARYLAND
Office of Licensure &
Certification Programs
Department of Health & Mental
Hygiene
4201 Patterson Avenue, 4th
Floor
Baltimore, MD 21215
(301) 764-2750

MASSACHUSETTS
Division of Health Care Quality
Department of Public Health
80 Boylston Street, Suite 1100
Boston, MA 02116
(617) 727-1296

MICHIGAN
Health Facilities Licensure &
Certification
Department of Public Health
3423 North Logan
P.O. Box 30195
Lansing, MI 48909
(517) 335-8505

MINNESOTA
Health Resources Division
Minnesota Department of Health
393 North Dunlap Street
St. Paul, MN 55164-0938
(612) 643-2100

MISSISSIPPI
Division of Licensure &
Certification
Health Care Commission
2688D Insurance Center Drive
Jackson, MS 39216
(601) 354-6645

MISSOURI
Division of Aging
Institutional Services Section
2701 West Main Street
Jefferson City, MO 65102
(314) 751-3082

MONTANA
Bureau of Licensure and
Certification
Division of Hospital and
Medical Facilities
Department of Health and
Environmental Science
Cogswell Building
Helena, MT 59620
(406) 444-2037

NEBRASKA
Department of Health
Division of Licensure & Standards
P.O. Box 95007
Lincoln, NE 68509
(402) 471-2946

NEVADA
Department of Health
Bureau of Regulatory Health
Services
505 East King Street, Room 202
Carson City, NV 89710
(702) 885-4475

NEW HAMPSHIRE
Division of Public Health
Services
Bureau of Health Facilities
Administration
Six Hazen Drive
Concord, NH 03301
(603) 271-4592

NEW JERSEY
Licensure Certification &
Standards
New Jersey Department of Health
CN367
Trenton, NJ 08625
(no phone listing)

NEW MEXICO
Health Facilities & Occupational
Licensure Bureau
Health Services Division
Health Environment Department
1190 St. Francis Drive
Santa Fe, NM 87501
(505) 827-2427

NEW YORK
Division of Health Center
Standards & Surveillance
Office of Health Systems
Management
State Department of Health
Tower Building, Room 1805
Empire State Plaza
Albany, NY 12237
(518) 473-3517

NORTH CAROLINA
Certification Section
Division of Facilities Services
701 Barbour Drive
Raleigh, NC 27603
(919) 733-7461

OHIO
Bureau of Medical Services
Ohio Department of Health
246 North High Street
P.O. Box 118
Columbus, OH 43266-0588
(614) 466-7857

OKLAHOMA
State Commission of Health
Department of Health
1000 NE 10th Street
Oklahoma City, OK 73152
(405) 271-4200

OREGON
Health Facilities Section
Health Division
1400 SW 5th Avenue, Room 605
Portland, OR 97207
(503) 229-5348

PENNSYLVANIA
Bureau of Quality Assurance
Pennsylvania Department of
Health
Health & Welfare Building,
Room 907
Harrisburg, PA 17120
(717) 787-8015

PUERTO RICO
Health & Service Facilities
Administration
Department of Health
P.O. Box 9312
Santurce, PR 00908
(809) 751-0531

RHODE ISLAND
Division of Facilities Regulation
Rhode Island Department of
Health
3 Capitol Hill, Room 306
Providence, RI 02908
(401) 277-2566

SOUTH CAROLINA
Division of Health, Licensure &
Certification
Department of Health &
Environmental Control
2600 Bull Street
Columbia, SC 29201
(803) 734-4680

SOUTH DAKOTA
Licensure & Certification
Program
South Dakota Department of
Health
523 East Capitol
Pierre, SD 57501
(605) 773-3364

TENNESSEE
Health Center Facilities
Department of Health &
Environment
283 Plus Park Boulevard
Nashville, TN 37217
(615) 367-6303

TEXAS
Quality Standards Division
Texas Department of Health
1100 West 49th Street
Austin, TX 78756
(512) 458-7611

UTAH
Facilities Survey Section
Division of Health Care
Financing
Department of Health
P.O. Box 16580
288 North, 1460 West
Salt Lake City, UT 84116-0580
(801) 538-6101

VERMONT
Long-Term Care Director
Vermont Department of Health
Box 70
Burlington, VT 05402
(802) 863-7250

VIRGINIA
Division of Medical & Nursing
Facilities Services
Department of Health
109 Governor Street
Richmond, VA 23219
(804) 786-2082

WASHINGTON
Aging & Adult Services
Administration
Department of Social & Health
Services
623 8th Avenue, SE
HB-11
Olympia, WA 98504-0095
(206) 753-5840

WEST VIRGINIA
Health Facilities Licensure &
Certification Division
West Virginia Department of
Health
1900 Kanawha Boulevard East
Building 3
Charleston, WV 25305
(304) 348-0050

WISCONSIN
Bureau of Quality Compliance
Wisconsin Division of Health
P.O. Box 309
Madison, WI 53701
(608) 267-7185

WYOMING
Division of Health & Medical
Services
Hathaway Building
2300 Capitol Avenue
Cheyenne, WY 82002-0710
(307) 777-7121

NURSING FACILITY LICENSE AND CERTIFICATION OFFICES

These offices are the government agencies in each state which inspect nursing facilities, issue state licenses and Medicare and Medicaid certifications. You can check the record of any nursing facility in the state through this office.

ALABAMA
Nursing Home Licensure Office
Division of Licensure and
Certification
Alabama Department of Health
434 Monroe Street
Montgomery, AL 36130
(205) 261-5113

ALASKA
Nursing Home Licensure Office
Department of Health and
Social Services
Health Facilities Certification
and Licensing
4433 Business Park Boulevard,
Building M
Anchorage, AK 99503
(907) 561-2171

ARIZONA
Department of Health Services
Office of Health Care Licensure
701 East Jefferson
Phoenix, AZ 85034
(602) 255-1177

ARKANSAS
Arkansas Department of Health
Certification and Licensure Section
Office of Long-Term Care
P.O. Box 8059, Slot 404
Little Rock, AR 72203
(501) 371-8143

CALIFORNIA
Nursing Home Licensure Office
Licensure and Certification
Division
Facilities Licensing Section
714 P Street, Room 823
Sacramento, CA 95814
(916) 445-3281

COLORADO
Nursing Home Licensure Office
Colorado Department of Health
Health Facilities Division
Evaluation and Licensure
Section
4210 East 11th Avenue, Room
254
Denver, CO 80220
(303) 331-4930

CONNECTICUT
Nursing Home Licensure Office
Connecticut State Department of
Health
Division of Hospital and
Medical Care
150 Washington Street
Hartford, CT 06106
(203) 566-5758

DELAWARE
Office of Health Facility
Licensing
and Certification
Nursing Home Division
Division of Public Health
3000 Newport Gap Pike
Wilmington, DE 19808
(302) 571-3499

DISTRICT OF COLUMBIA
Office of Licensing and
Certification
Nursing Home Division
Department of Human Services
614 H Street, NW, Suite 1014
Washington, DC 20001
(202) 727-7190

FLORIDA
Nursing Home Licensure Office
Licensure and Certification
Branch
Division of Health
Department of Rehabilitation
Services
2727 Mahan Drive
Tallahassee, FL 32308
(904) 487-3513

GEORGIA
Nursing Home Licensure Office
Standards and Licensure Unit
Office of Regulatory Services
878 Peachtree Street, NE
Suite 803
Atlanta, GA 30309
(404) 894-5137

HAWAII
Nursing Home Licensure Office
Hospital and Medical Facility
Branch
Hawaii State Department of
Health
P.O. Box 3378
Honolulu, HI 96801
(808) 548-5935

IDAHO
Nursing Home Licensure Office
Facilities Standards and
Development
Idaho Department of Health and
Welfare
450 West State Street, 2nd Floor
Boise, ID 83720
(208) 334-6626

ILLINOIS
Nursing Home Licensure Office
Illinois Department of Public
Health
Health Facilities and Quality of
Care
525 West Jefferson, Fifth Floor
Springfield, IL 62761
(217) 782-5180

INDIANA
Nursing Home Licensure Office
Division of Health Facilities
Indiana State Board of Health
1330 West Michigan Street,
Room 336
P.O. Box 1964
Indianapolis, IN 46206-1964
(317) 633-8442

IOWA
Nursing Home Licensure Office
State Department of Inspections
& Appeals
Division of Health Facilities
Lucas State Office Building, 3rd
Floor
Des Moines, IA 50319
(515) 281-4115

KANSAS
Kansas Department of Health
and Environment
Bureau of Adult and Child Care
Landon State Office Building
900 SW Jackson, Suite 1001
Topeka, KS 66612-1290
(913) 296-1240

KENTUCKY
Nursing Home Licensure Office
Division for Licensing and
Regulation
CHR Building, Fourth Floor East
275 East Main Street
Frankfort, KY 40621-0001
(502) 564-2800

LOUISIANA
Nursing Home Licensure Office
Department of Health and
Human Resources
Division of Licensure &
Certification
P.O. Box 3767
Baton Rouge, LA 70821-3767
(504) 342-5774

MAINE
Nursing Home Licensure Office
Division of Licensure and
Certification
249 Western Avenue
State House Station 11
Augusta, ME 04333
(207) 289-2606

MARYLAND
Office of Licensing and
Certification Program
Department of Health and
Mental Hygiene
4201 Patterson Avenue, 4th
Floor
Baltimore, MD 21215
(301) 764-2750

MASSACHUSETTS
Nursing Home Licensure Office
Long-Term Care Facilities
Program
Department of Public Health
80 Boylston Street, Eleventh
Floor
Boston, MA 02116
(617) 727-5864

MICHIGAN
Nursing Home Licensure Office
Bureau of Health Care
Administration
Department of Public Health
3423 North Logan Street
P.O. Box 30195
Lansing, MI 48909
(517) 335-8505

MINNESOTA
Nursing Home Licensure Office
Minnesota Department of Health
Survey and Compliance Section
393 North Dunlap Street
P.O. Box 64900
St. Paul, MN 55164-0900
(612) 643-2101

MISSISSIPPI
Nursing Home Licensure Office
Health Facilities Certification
and Licensure
Mississippi State Board of
Health
2423 North State Street
P.O. Box 1700
Jackson, MS 39215-1700
(601) 960-7769

MISSOURI
Missouri Department of Social
Services
Division of Aging
P.O. Box 1337
1440 Aaron Court
Jefferson City, MO 65102
(314) 751-2712

MONTANA
Montana Department of Health
and Environmental Sciences
Bureau of Licensing and
Certification
Health Services Division
Cogswell Building
Helena, MT 59620
(406) 444-2037

NEBRASKA
Division of Licensure and
Standards
Nursing Home Division
Department of Health
301 Centennial Mall South
P.O. Box 95007
Lincoln, NE 68509
(402) 471-2946

NEVADA
Nursing Home Licensure Office
Bureau of Regulatory Health
Services
505 East King Street, Room 202
Carson City, NV 89710
(702) 885-4475

NEW HAMPSHIRE
Department of Health and
Human Services
Division of Public Health
Bureau of Health Facilities
Administration
Six Hazen Drive
Concord, NH 03301-6527
(603) 271-4592

NEW JERSEY
Nursing Home Licensure Office
New Jersey State Department of
Health
Licensing, Certification and
Standards
300 Whitehead Road
Trenton, NJ 08625
(609) 588-7725

NEW MEXICO
Nursing Home Licensure Office
Health and Social Services
Department
4125 Carlisle, NE
Albuquerque, NM 87107
(505) 841-6524

NEW YORK
Bureau of Long-Term Care
Services
Corning, Second Tower
Empire State Plaza, 18th Floor
Albany, NY 12237
(518) 473-1564

NORTH CAROLINA
Nursing Home Licensure Office
Licensure and Certification
Section
Health Care Facilities Branch
701 Barbour Drive
Raleigh, NC 27603
(919) 733-2786

NORTH DAKOTA
Division of Health Facilities
State Department of Health
Nursing Home Division
State Capitol, Judicial Wing
600 East Boulevard Avenue
Bismarck, ND 58505
(701) 224-2352

OHIO
Nursing Home Licensure Office
Medical Services
Licensing and Certification
Division
Ohio Department of Health
246 North High Street
Box 118
Columbus, OH 43266-0118
(614) 466-2070

OKLAHOMA
Nursing Home Licensure Office
Licensure and Certification
Division
Oklahoma State Department of
Health
1000 NE Tenth
P.O. Box 53551, Fourth Floor
Oklahoma City, OK 73152
(405) 271-5116

OREGON
Senior Services Division
Long-Term Care Licensing
Licensing and Certification
313 Public Service Building
Salem, OR 97310
(503) 378-3751

PENNSYLVANIA
Nursing Home Licensure Office
Commonwealth of Pennsylvania
Division of Long-Term Care
Health and Welfare Building
Room 526
Harrisburg, PA 17120
(717) 787-1816

RHODE ISLAND
Nursing Home Licensure Office
Rhode Island Department of
Health
Division of Facilities Regulation
3 Capitol Hill
Providence, RI 02908-5097
(401) 277-2566

SOUTH CAROLINA
Nursing Home Licensure Office
Division of Health Facilities and
Services
Department of Health Licensing
2600 Bull Street
Columbia, SC 29201
(803) 734-4680

SOUTH DAKOTA
Department of Health
Division of Licensure and
Certification
523 East Capitol Street
Pierre, SD 57501-3182
(605) 773-3364

TENNESSEE
Department of Health and
Environment
Board for Licensing Health Care
Facilities
283 Plus Park Boulevard
Nashville, TN 37219-5407
(615) 367-6303

TEXAS
Nursing Home Licensure Office
Texas Department of Health
Quality Standards Division
1100 West 49th Street, Room
202
Austin, TX 78756-3199
(512) 458-7490

UTAH
Nursing Home Licensure Office
Utah Department of Health
Bureau of Health Facilities
Licensing
P.O. Box 16660
Salt Lake City, UT 84116-0660
(801) 538-6152

VERMONT
Nursing Home Licensure Office
Vermont Department of Health
Medical Regulation
19 Commerce Street, Box 536
Williston, VT 05495
(802) 863-7250

VIRGINIA
Nursing Home Licensure Office
Division of Licensure and
Certification
1013 Madison Building
109 Governor Street
Richmond, VA 23219
(804) 786-2081

WASHINGTON
Nursing Home Licensure Office
DSHS-Health Services Division
Aging and Adult Services
Administration
623 8th Avenue, SE
Mail Stop HB-11
Olympia, WA 98504
(206) 753-5840

WEST VIRGINIA
Nursing Home Licensure Office
Health Facilities and
Certification Section
1900 Kanawha Boulevard East
Building 3, Room 535
Charleston, WV 25305
(304) 348-0050

WISCONSIN
Department of Health and Social
Services
Division of Health
Bureau of Quality Compliance
One West Wilson Street
Room 150, P.O. Box 309
Madison, WI 53701
(608) 266-3024

WYOMING
Department of Health and Social
Services
Division of Health and Medical
Services
Medical Facilities
Hathaway Building, Fourth
Floor
Cheyenne, WY 82002-0717
(307) 777-7121

OMBUDSMAN OFFICES

Most states have a central office that can refer you to the long-term care ombudsman nearest you. The long-term care ombudsman responds to complaints about abuse at long-term care facilities and can mediate disputes between residents and the facilities. There is no charge for their services.

ALABAMA
Commission on Aging
136 Catoma Street
Montgomery, AL 36130
(205) 242-5743

ALASKA
Older Alaskans Ombudsman
3601 C Street, Suite 260
Anchorage, AK 99503
(907) 279-2232

ARIZONA
Aging and Adult Administration
1400 West Washington Street
Phoenix, AZ 85007
(602) 542-4446

ARKANSAS
Office on Aging and Adult
Services
Department of Human Services
1417 Donaghey
7th and Main Streets
P.O. Box 1437
Little Rock, AR 72203
(501) 682-2441

CALIFORNIA
California Department on Aging
1600 K Street
Sacramento, CA 95814
(916) 323-6681

COLORADO
Medical Care & Research
Foundation
1420 Ogden
Denver, CO 80218
(303) 831-0267

CONNECTICUT
Connecticut Department on
Aging
221 Main Street
Hartford, CT 06106
(203) 566-7770

DELAWARE
Division on Aging
Milford State Service Center
11-13 Church Avenue
Milford, DE 19963
(302) 422-1386

**DISTRICT OF
COLUMBIA**
Legal Counsel for the Elderly
1909 K Street, NW
Washington, DC 20039
(202) 662-4933

FLORIDA
State Long-Term Care
Ombudsman Committee
Department of Health
and Rehabilitative Services
Building 1, #308
1317 Winewood Boulevard
Tallahassee, FL 32399-0700
(904) 488-6190

GEORGIA
Office of Aging
Department of Human
Resources
2719 Buford Highway, NE
Atlanta, GA 30324
(404) 728-0223

HAWAII
Hawaii Executive Office on
Aging
335 Merchant Street, Suite 241
Honolulu, HI 96813
(808) 548-2593

IDAHO
Idaho Office on Aging
State House, Room 108
Boise, ID 83720
(208) 334-3833

ILLINOIS
Department on Aging
421 East Capitol Avenue
Springfield, IL 62701
(217) 785-3371

INDIANA
Indiana Department of Human
Services
Aging Services Division
251 North Illinois
P.O. Box 7083
Indianapolis, IN 46207-7083
(317) 232-7115

IOWA
Iowa Department of Elder
Affairs
Jewett Building, Suite 236
914 Grand Avenue
Des Moines, IA 50319
(515) 281-5187

KANSAS
Department on Aging
915 SW Harrison
Docking State Office Building,
Room 122 South
Topeka, KS 66612
(913) 296-4986

KENTUCKY
Division for Aging Services
Department of Human
Resources
275 East Main Street, 6th Floor
West
Frankfort, KY 40621
(502) 564-6930

LOUISIANA
Governor's Office of Elderly
Affairs
4550 North Boulevard, 2nd
Floor
Baton Rouge, LA 70806
(504) 925-1700

MAINE
Maine Committee on Aging
State House Station 127
Augusta, ME 04333
(207) 289-3658

MARYLAND
Maryland Office on Aging
301 West Preston Street, Room
1004
Baltimore, MD 21201
(301) 225-1100

MASSACHUSETTS
Massachusetts Executive Office
of Elder Affairs
38 Chauncy Street
Boston, MA 02111
(617) 727-7273

MICHIGAN
Citizens for Better care
1627 East Kalamazoo
Lansing, MI 48917
(517) 482-1297

MINNESOTA
Minnesota Board on Aging
444 Lafayette Road
St. Paul, MN 55155-3843
(612) 296-7465

MISSISSIPPI
Mississippi Council on Aging
421 West Pascagoula Street
Jackson, MS 39201
(601) 949-2070

MISSOURI
Division on Aging
Department of Social Services
2701 West Main
Jefferson City, MO 65102
(314) 751-3082

MONTANA
Governor's Office on Aging
Capitol Station
Helena, MT 59620
(406) 444-4202

NEBRASKA
Department on Aging
P.O. Box 95044
Lincoln, NE 68509
(402) 471-2307

NEVADA
Divison of Aging Services
Department of Human
Resources
1665 Hot Springs, Suite 158
Carson City, NV 89710

NEW HAMPSHIRE
Division of Elderly Services
Six Hazen Drive
Concord, NH 03301
(603) 271-4680

NEW JERSEY
Office of the Ombudsman
for the Institutionalized Elderly
Room 305, CN808
28 West State Street
Trenton, NJ 08625-0808
(609) 292-8016

NEW MEXICO
State Agency on Aging
LaVilla Rivera Building, 4th Floor
224 East Palace Avenue
Santa Fe, NM 87501
(505) 827-7640

NEW YORK
Office for the Aging
Agency Building #2
Empire State Plaza
Albany, NY 12223
(518) 474-5731

NORTH CAROLINA
North Carolina Department
of Human Resources
Division of Aging
693 Palmer Drive
Raleigh, NC 27603
(919) 733-3983

NORTH DAKOTA
Aging Services Division
Department of Human Services
600 East Boulevard
Bismarck, ND 58505
(701) 224-2577

OHIO
Ohio Department on Aging
50 West Broad Street, 9th Floor
Columbus, OH 43266-0501
(614) 466-9927

OKLAHOMA
State Long-Term Care
Ombudsperson
Aging Services
P.O. Box 25352
Oklahoma City, OK 73125

OREGON
Office of Long-Term Care
Ombudsman
2475 Lancaster Drive, NE
Building B, #9
Salem, OR 97310
(503) 378-6533

PENNSYLVANIA
Department of Aging
231 State Street
Harrisburg, PA 17101
(717) 783-7247

PUERTO RICO
Gericulture Commission
Department of Social Services
G.P.O. Box 11398
Santurce, PR 00910
(809) 722-7400

RHODE ISLAND
Rhode Island Department
of Elderly Affairs
160 Pine Street
Providence, RI 02903
(401) 277-6880

SOUTH CAROLINA
Office of the Governor
Divison of Ombudsman
and Citizens' Services
1205 Pendleton Street, Suite 308
Columbia, SC 29201
(803) 734-0457

SOUTH DAKOTA
Office of Adult Services and
Aging
Department of Social Services
700 Governor's Drive
Pierre, SD 57501-2291
(605) 773-3656

TENNESSEE
Commission on Aging
706 Church Street, Suite 201
Nashville, TN 37219
(615) 741-2056

TEXAS
Texas Department on Aging
P.O. Box 12786 Capitol Station
Austin, TX 78711
(512) 444-2727

UTAH
Division of Aging and Adult
Services
Department of Social Services
120 North, 200 West, Room 401
Salt Lake City, UT 84103
(801) 538-3910

VERMONT
Vermont Office on Aging
103 South Main Street
Waterbury, VT 05676
(802) 241-2400

VIRGINIA
Department for the Aging
700 East Franklin Street
10th Floor
Richmond, VA 23219

WASHINGTON
Multi-Service Center
1200 South 336
Federal Way, WA 98003

WEST VIRGINIA
Commission on Aging
State Capitol Complex
Charleston, WV 25305
(304) 348-3317

WISCONSIN
Board on Aging and
Long-Term Care
819 North 6th, Room 619
Milwaukee, WI 53203-1664
(414) 227-4386

WYOMING
Long-Term Care
Ombudsman Program
P.O. Box 94
Wheatland, WY 82201

RESIDENTIAL REFERRALS

NURSING FACILITY AND ALTERNATIVE RESIDENCE ORGANIZATIONS

American Association of Homes for the Aging
1129 20th Street, NW
Washington, DC 20036
(202) 296-5960

AAHA is a national association of non-profit-only nursing facilities and senior independent living centers. It will provide a list of all member facilities in your state, including level of facility, type of sponsorship, number of living units or beds and community services offered to non-residents.

American Health Care Association
12301 L Street, NW
Washington, DC 20005
(202) 842-4444

AHCA is a national association of both profit and non-profit accredited nursing facilities. It will provide a list of its member facilities in your state.

Joseph Matthews has been an attorney since 1971, and from 1975 to 1977 he taught at the law school of the University of California, Berkeley. He has for many years been involved in matters relating to seniors, and is the author of *Social Security, Medicare & Pensions: The Sourcebook for Older Americans* (Nolo Press), now in its 5th edition.

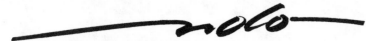

FAMILY MATTERS

A Legal Guide for Lesbian and Gay Couples

ATTORNEYS HAYDEN CURRY & DENIS CLIFFORD
NATIONAL 5TH ED.

Laws designed to regulate and protect married couples don't apply to lesbian and gay couples. This book shows you, step-by-step, how to write a living-together contract, plan for medical emergencies (using durable powers of attorney), and plan your estates (wills and probate avoidance techniques). It also discusses legal aspects of having and raising children and relating to ex-spouses and children of former marriages. Complete with forms, sample agreements and lists of both national lesbian and gay legal organizations, and AIDS organizations.

$17.95 / LG

The Guardianship Book

BY LISA GOLDOFTAS &
ATTORNEY DAVID BROWN
CALIFORNIA 1ST ED.

Thousands of children in California are left without a guardian because their parents have died, abandoned them or are unable to care for them. *The Guardianship Book* provides step-by-step instructions and the forms needed to obtain a legal guardianship without a lawyer.

$19.95 / GB

How to Do Your Own Divorce

ATTORNEY CHARLES E. SHERMAN
(TEXAS ED. BY SHERMAN & SIMONS)
CALIFORNIA 15TH ED. & TEXAS 2ND ED.

This is the book that launched Nolo Press and advanced the self-help law movement. During the past 18 years, over 500,000 copies have been sold, saving consumers at least $50 million in legal fees (assuming 100,000 have each saved $500—certainly a conservative estimate). Contains all the forms and instructions you need to do your divorce without a lawyer.

CALIFORNIA $18.95 / CDIV
TEXAS $14.95 / TDIV

Practical Divorce Solutions

ATTORNEY CHARLES E. SHERMAN
CALIFORNIA 1ST ED.

This book is a valuable guide to the emotional aspects of divorce as well as an overview of the legal and financial decisions that must be made.

$12.95 / PDS

The Living Together Kit

ATTORNEYS TONI IHARA & RALPH WARNER
NATIONAL 6TH ED.

"Written in plain language, free of legal mumbo jumbo, and spiced with witty personal observations."

—**Associated Press**

The Living Together Kit is a detailed guide designed to help the increasing number of unmarried couples living together understand the laws that affect them. *The Living Together Kit* contains comprehensive information on estate planning, paternity agreements, living together agreements, buying real estate, and much more. Sample agreements and instructions are included.

$17.95 / LTK

How to Adopt You Stepchild in California

FRANK ZAGONE & ATTORNEY MARY RANDOLPH
CALIFORNIA 3RD ED.

For many families that include stepchildren, adoption is a sure-fire way to avoid confusion over inheritance or guardianship. This book provides sample forms and complete step-by-step instructions for completing a simple uncontested stepparent adoption in California.

$19.95 / ADOP

How to Modify and Collect Child Support In California

ATTORNEYS JOSEPH MATTHEWS, WARREN SIEGEL & MARY WILLIS
CALIFORNIA 3RD ED.

Using this book, parents can determine the level of child support they are entitled to receive, or obliged to pay, and can go to court to modify existing support to the appropriate level.

$17.95 / SUPP

California Marriage & Divorce Law

ATTORNEYS RALPH WARNER, TONI IHARA & STEPHEN ELIAS
CALIFORNIA 10TH ED.

This practical handbook is for the Californian who wants to understand marriage and divorce laws. It explains community property, pre-nuptial contracts, foreign marriages, buying a house, the steps for getting a divorce, dividing property, and much more.

$17.95 / MARR

PATENT, COPYRIGHT & TRADEMARK

Patent it Yourself

ATTORNEY DAVID PRESSMAN
NATIONAL 2ND ED.

Every step of the patent process is presented in order in this gem of a book, complete with official forms..."

—**San Francisco Chronicle**

This state-of-the-art guide is a must for all inventors interested in obtaining patents—from the patent search to the actual application. Patent attorney and former patent examiner David Pressman covers use and licensing, successful marketing, and how to deal with infringement.

$29.95 / PAT

The Inventor's Notebook

GRISSOM & ATTORNEY PRESSMAN
NATIONAL 1ST ED.

The best protection for your patent is adequate records. *The Inventor's Notebook* helps you document the process of successful independent inventing by provideing forms, instructions, references to relevant areas of patent law, a bibliography of legal and non-legal aids, and more.

$19.95 / INOT

How to Copyright Software

ATTORNEY M.J. SALONE
NATIONAL 3RD ED.

"Written by practicing lawyers in the straightforward and informative Nolo style, the book covers just about everything that might be of interest to a software developer or publisher. Even those who are employed by a company on a full-time or contractual basis will find much to ponder here."

—**PC Week**

Now that you've spent hours of time and sleepless nights perfecting your software creation, learn how to protect it from plagiarism. Copyright laws give you rights against those who use your work without your permission. This book tells you how to enforce those rights, how to register your copyright for maximum protection, and discusses who owns a copyright on software developed by more than one person.

$34.95 / COPY

Legal Care for Your Software

ATTORNEYS DANIEL REMER & STEPHEN ELIAS
NATIONAL

Legal Care for Your Software is out of print. Nolo authors are in the process of writing a new 4th edition of this book.

BUSINESS

The Independent Paralegal's Handbook

ATTORNEY RALPH WARNER
NATIONAL 1ST ED.
A large percentage of routine legal work in this country is performed by typists, secretaries, researchers and other law office helpers generally labeled paralegals. For those who want to take these services out of the law office and offer them for a reasonable fee in an independent business, attorney Ralph Warner provides legal and business guidelines.
$12.95 / PARA

Getting Started as an Independent Paralegal

(TWO AUDIO TAPES)
ATTORNEY RALPH WARNER
NATIONAL 1ST ED.
Approximately three hours in all, these tapes are a carefully edited version of a seminar given by Nolo Press founder Ralph Warner. They are designed to be used with *The Independent Paralegal's Handbook.*
$24.95 / GSIP

Marketing Without Advertising

MICHAEL PHILLIPS & SALLI RASBERRY
NATIONAL 1ST ED.
"There are good ideas on every page. You'll find here the nitty gritty steps you need to—and can—take to generate sales for your business, no matter what business it is."

—Milton Moskowitz, syndicated columnist and author of The 100 Best Companies to Work For in America

The best marketing plan encourages customer loyalty and personal recommendation. Phillips and Rasberry outline practical steps for building and expanding a small business without spending a lot of money on advertising.
$14.00 / MWA

The Partnership Book

ATTORNEYS CLIFFORD & WARNER
NATIONAL 3RD ED.
Lots of people dream of going into business with a friend. The best way to keep that dream from turning into a nightmare is to have a solid partnership agreement. This book shows you, step-by-step, how to write an agreement that meets your need. It covers initial contributions to the business, wages, profit-sharing, buy-outs, death or retirement of a partner, and disputes.
$18.95 / PART

How to Write a Business Plan

MIKE MCKEEVER
NATIONAL 3RD ED.
"...outlines the kinds of credit available... shows how to prepare cashflow forecasts, capital spending plans, and other vital ideas. An attractive guide for would-be entrepreneurs."

—ALA Booklist

If you're thinking of starting a business or raising money to expand an existing one, this book will show you how to write the business plan and loan package necessary to finance your business and make it work.
$17.95 / SBS

How to Form Your Own Corporation

ATTORNEY ANTHONY MANCUSO
CALIFORNIA 7TH ED.
TEXAS 4TH ED.
NEW YORK 2ND ED.
FLORIDA 2ND ED.
Incorporating your small business lets you take advantage of tax benefits, limited liability and benefits of employee status, and financial flexibility. These books contain the forms, instructions and tax information you need to incorporate a small business yourself and save hundreds of dollars in lawyers' fees. Each contains up-to-date corporate and tax information.
CALIFORNIA $29.95 / CCOR
TEXAS $24.95 / TCOR
NEW YORK $24.95 / NYCO
FLORIDA $24.95 / FLCO

The California Professional Corporation Handbook

ATTORNEY ANTHONY MANCUSO
CALIFORNIA 4TH ED.
Health care professionals, lawyers, accountants and members of certain other professions must fulfill special requirements when forming a corporation in California. Professional corporations offer liability protection, the financial benefits of a corporate retirement plan, and lower tax rates on the first $75,000 of taxable income. This edition contains up-to-date tax information plus all the forms and instructions necessary to form a California professional corporation. An appendix explains the special rules that apply to each profession.
$34.95 / PROF

The California Nonprofit Corporation Handbook

ATTORNEY ANTHONY MANCUSO
CALIFORNIA 5TH ED.
Tthis book shows you step-by-step how to form and operate a nonprofit corporation in California. It includes the latest corporate and tax law changes, including expanded protection from personal liability for corporate directors. Includes forms for the Articles, Bylaws and Minutes you need. Contains complete instructions for obtaining federal 501(c)(3) tax exemptions and benefits, which may be used in any state.
$29.95 / NON

OLDER AMERICANS

Elder Care: Choosing and Financing Long-Term Care

JOSEPH L. MATTHEWS
NATIONAL 1ST ED.
Until recently, the only choice for the elderly in deteriorating health was to enter a nursing home. Now older people who need care and their families are faced with many more choices, ranging from care at home to residential facilities to complete care homes. This book will guide you in choosing and paying for long-term care, alerting you to practical concerns and explaining laws that may affect your decisions.
$16.95 / ELD

Social Security, Medicare & Pensions

ATTORNEY JOSEPH MATTHEWS & DOROTHY MATTHEWS BERMAN
NATIONAL 5TH ED.
When the Catastrophic Coverage Act was repealed recently, it drastically changed the kinds and amounts of government benefits for older Americans. While assistance with income and healthcare is still available, it requires more perseverance and understanding to get your due.

This new edition includes invaluable guidance through the current maze of rights and benefits for those 55 and over, including Medicare, Medicaid and Social Security retirement and disability benefits and age discrimination protections.
$15.95 / SOA

ESTATE PLANNING & PROBATE

Plan Your Estate

ATTORNEY DENIS CLIFFORD
NATIONAL 1ST ED.

"One of the best personal finance books of 1989." —Money Magazine

This book overs every significant aspect of estate planning, and gives detailed, specific instructions for preparing a living trust. *Plan Your Estate* shows how to prepare an estate plan without the expensive services of a lawyer and ncludes all the tear-out forms and step-by-step instructions to let people with estates under $600,000 do the job themselves.

$17.95 / NEST

Nolo's Simple Will Book

ATTORNEY DENIS CLIFFORD
NATIONAL 2ND ED.

It's easy to write a legally valid will using this book. The instructions and forms enable people to draft a will for all needs, including naming a personal guardian for minor children; leaving property to minor children or young adults; and updating a will when necessary. This edition also contains a discussion of estate planning basics with information on living trusts, death taxes, and durable powers of attorney. Good in all states except Louisiana.

$17.95 / SWIL

How To Probate an Estate

JULIA NISSLEY
CALIFORNIA 5TH ED.

If you find yourself responsible for winding up the legal and financial affairs of a deceased family member or friend, you can often save costly attorneys' fees by handling the probate process yourself. *How to Probate an Estate* shows you, step-by-step, how to actually settle an estate. It also covers the simple procedures you can use to transfer assets that don't require probate, including property held in joint tenancy or living trusts or as community property.

$24.95 / PAE

The Power of Attorney Book

ATTORNEY DENIS CLIFFORD
NATIONAL 3RD ED.

Who will take care of your affairs, and make your financial and medical decisions if you can't? With *The Power of Attorney Book* you can appoint someone you trust to carry out your wishes and stipulate exactly what kind of care you want or don't want. Includes Durable Power of Attorney and Living Will forms.

$19.95 / POA

GOING TO COURT

Everybody's Guide to Small Claims Court

ATTORNEY RALPH WARNER
NATIONAL 4TH ED.
CALIFORNIA 8TH ED.

So, the dry cleaner ruined your good flannel suit. Your roof leaks every time it rains, and the contractor who supposedly fixed it won't call you back. The landlord won't return your security deposit. This book will help you decide if you should sue in small claims court, show you how to file and serve papers, tell you what to bring to court, and how to collect a judgment.

NATIONAL $14.95 / NSCC
CALIFORNIA $14.95 / CSCC

Collect Your Court Judgment

GINI GRAHAM SCOTT, ATTORNEY STEPHEN ELIAS & LISA GOLDOFTAS
CALIFORNIA 1ST ED.

After you win a judgment in small claims, municipal or superior court, you still have to collect your money. If the debtor doesn't pay up voluntarily, you need to know how to collect your judgment from the debtor's bank accounts, wages, business receipts, real estate or other assets. This book contains step-by-step instructions and all the forms you need.

$24.95 / JUDG

Fight Your Ticket

ATTORNEY DAVID BROWN
CALIFORNIA 3RD ED.

Here's a book that shows you how to fight an unfair traffic ticket—when you're stopped, at arraignment, at trial and on appeal. No wonder a traffic court judge (who must remain nameless) told us that he keeps this book by his bench for easy reference!

$16.95 / FYT

The Criminal Records Book

ATTORNEY WARREN SIEGEL
CALIFORNIA 3RD ED.

We've all done something illegal. If you were one of those who got caught, your juvenile or criminal court record can complicate your life years later. The good news is that in many cases your record can either be completely expunged or lessened in severity. *The Criminal Records Book* shows you, step-by-step, how to seal criminal records, dismiss convictions, destroy marijuana records, and reduce felony convictions.

$19.95 / CRIM

Dog Law

ATTORNEY MARY RANDOLPH
NATIONAL 1ST ED.

Do you own a dog? Do you live down the street from one? If you do, you need *Dog Law*, a practical guide to the laws that affect dog owners and their neighbors. *Dog Law* answers common questions on such topics as biting, barking, veterinarians, leash laws, travel, landlords, wills, guide dogs, pit bulls, cruelty and much more.

$12.95 / DOG

How to Change Your Name

ATTORNEYS DAVID LOEB & DAVID BROWN
CALIFORNIA 4TH ED.

Wish you had gone back to your former name after the divorce? Tired of spelling V-e-n-k-a-t-a-r-a-m-a-n S-u-b-r-a-m-a-n-i-a-m over the phone? This book explains how to change your name legally and provides all the necessary court forms with detailed instructions on how to fill them out.

$19.95 / NAME

MONEY MATTERS

How to File For Bankruptcy

ATTORNEYS STEPHEN ELIAS, ALBIN RENAUER & ROBIN LEONARD
NATIONAL 1ST ED.

It's no fun having to think about declaring bankruptcy. But easy credit, high interest rates, unexpected illness, job lay-offs and inflation often conspire to leave people with a satchel full of debts. Here we show you how to decide whether or not filing for bankruptcy makes sense and if it does, we give you forms and step-by-step instructionson how to do it.

$24.95 / HFB

Simple Contracts for Personal Use

ATTORNEY STEPHEN ELIAS
NATIONAL 1ST ED.

If you've ever sold a car, lent money to a relative or friend, or put money down on a prospective purchase, you should have used a contract. Perhaps everything went without a hitch. If it didn't, you probably experienced a lot of grief and frustration.

Here are clearly written legal form contracts to: buy and sell property, borrow and lend money, store and lend personal property, make deposits on goods for later purchase, release others from personal liability, or pay a contractor to do home repairs.

$12.95 / CONT

Homestead Your House

ATTORNEYS RALPH WARNER, CHARLES SHERMAN
& TONI IHARA
CALIFORNIA 7TH ED.

Under California homestead laws, up to
$75,000 of the equity in your home may be
safe from creditors. But to get the maximum legal protection, you should file a
Declaration of Homestead before a credi-
tor gets a court judgment against you and
puts a lien (legal claim) on your house.
This book shows you how and includes
complete instructions and tear-out forms.
$9.95 / HOME

The Deeds Book

ATTORNEY MARY RANDOLPH
CALIFORNIA 1ST ED.

If you own real estate, you'll need to sign a
new deed when you transfer the property
or put it in trust as part of your estate
planning. *The Deeds Book* shows you how
to choose the right kind of deed, complete
the tear-out forms, and record them in the
county recorder's public records. It also
alerts you to real property disclosure requirements and California community
property rules, as well as tax and estate
planning aspects of property transfers.
$15.95 / DEED

For Sale by Owner

GEORGE DEVINE
CALIFORNIA 1ST ED.

If you sell your house at California's me-
dian price—$200,000—the standard
broker's commission (6%) amounts to
$12,000. That's money you could save if
you sold your own house. This book provides essential information about pricing
your house, marketing it, writing a contract and going through escrow. With *For
Sale by Owner*, you can do the job yourself
and with confidence. Disclosure and contract forms are included.
$24.95 / FSBO

The Landlord's Law Book: Vol. 1, Rights & Responsibilities

ATTORNEYS DAVID BROWN & RALPH WARNER
CALIFORNIA 2ND ED.

The era when a landlord could substitute
common sense for a detailed knowledge of
the law is gone forever. Everything from the
amount you can charge for a security deposit to terminating a tenancy, to your legal
responsibility for the illegal acts of your
manager is closely regulated by the law.
This volume covers: deposits, leases and
rental agreements, inspections (tenants'
privacy rights), habitability (rent with-
holding), ending a tenancy, liability, and
rent control.
$24.95 / LBRT

The Landlord's Law Book: Vol. 2, Evictions

ATTORNEY DAVID BROWN
CALIFORNIA 2ND ED.

What do you do if you've got a tenant who
won't pay the rent—and won't leave?
There's only one choice: go to court and get
an eviction. This book takes you through
the process step-by-step. It's even got a special section on local rent control laws. All
the tear-out forms and instructions you
need are included.
$24.95 / LBEV

Tenants' Rights

ATTORNEYS MYRON MOSKOVITZ &
RALPH WARNER
CALIFORNIA 10TH ED.

Your "security building" doesn't have a
working lock on the front door. Is your
landlord liable? How can you get him to fix
it? Under what circumstances can you
withhold rent? When is an apartment not
"habitable?" Moskovitz and Warner explain the best way to handle your relationship with your landlord and your legal
rights when you find yourself in disagree-
ment. A special section on rent control
cities is included.
$15.95 / CTEN

Legal Research

ATTORNEY STEPHEN ELIAS
NATIONAL 2ND ED.

A valuable tool on its own, or as a companion to just about every other Nolo book.
Legal Research gives easy-to-use, step-by-
step instructions on how to find legal information. The legal self-helper can find and
research a case, read statutes and administrative regulations, and make Freedom of
Information Act requests. A great resource
for paralegals, law students, legal secretaries
and social workers.
$14.95 / LRES

Family Law Dictionary

ATTORNEYS ROBIN LEONARD & STEPHEN ELIAS
NATIONAL 1ST ED.

Finally, a legal dictionary that's written in
plain English, not "legalese"! The *Family
Law Dictionary* is designed to help the
nonlawyer who has a question or problem
involving family law—marriage, divorce,
adoption, or living together. The book
contains many examples as well as definitions, and extensive cross-references to
help you find the information you need.
$13.95 / FLD

Patent, Copyright & Trademark: The Intellectual Property Law Dictionary

ATTORNEY STEPHEN ELIAS
NATIONAL 1ST ED.

*...uses simple language free of legal jargon to
define and explain the intricacies of items associated with trade secrets, copyrights, trade-
marks and unfair competition, patents and
patent procedures, and contracts and warran-
ties.*

—IEEE Spectrum

If you're dealing with any multi-media
product, a new business product or trade
secret, you need this book.
$19.95 / IPLD

WillMaker

NOLO PRESS & LEGISOFT, INC.
NATIONAL 3RD ED.

"A well crafted document. That's even what my lawyer said …noting that a few peculiar twists in my state's law were handled nicely by the computerized lawyer."

—Peter H. Lewis, The New York Times

"An excellent addition to anyone's home-productivity library."

—Home Office Computing

"A fertile hybrid that I expect to see more of: can-do software that lives inside a how-to-book. In this case, the book itself is one of the better ones on preparing your own will."

—Whole Earth Review

Recent statistics say chances are better than 2 to 1 that you haven't written a will, even though you know you should. *WillMaker* makes the job easy, leading you step-by-step in a question and answer format. Once you've gone through the program, you print out the will and sign it in front of witnesses. Because writing a will is only one step in the estate planning process, *WillMaker* comes with a 200-page manual providing an overview of probate avoidance and tax planning techniques. Good in all states except Louisiana.

APPLE II	$59.95	WA3
IBM PC 3 1/2	$59.95	W3I3
IBM PC 5 1/4	$59.95	WI3
MACINTOSH	$59.95	WM3
MACINTOSH 512K	$59.95	WM3K

For the Record

CAROL PLADSEN & ATTORNEY RALPH WARNER
NATIONAL 1ST ED.

This easy-to-use software program provides a single place to keep a complete inventory of all your important legal, financial, personal, and family records. Having accurate and complete records facilitates tax preparation and helps loved ones manage your affairs if you become incapacitated or die. The detailed manual offers an overview of how to reduce estate taxes and avoid probate, and tells you what records you need to keep.

MACINTOSH	$49.95	FRM
IBM PC 3 1/2	$49.95	FR3I
IBM PC 5 1/4	$49.95	FRI

California Incorporator

ATTORNEY ANTHONY MANCUSO & LEGISOFT, INC.
CALIFORNIA 1ST ED.

"…easy to use…the manual consists of far more than instructions for using the software…[it is] a primer that provides a great deal of background, including detailed explanations of the legal implications of each decision you make."

—Los Angeles Times

About half of the small California corporations formed today are done without the services of a lawyer. Now, this easy-to-use software program makes the job even easier.

Just answer the questions on the screen, and *California Incorporator* will print out the 35-40 pages of documents you need to make your California corporation legal.

Comes with a 200-page manual that explains the incorporation process.

IBM PC 3 1/2	$129.00	INCI
IBM PC 5 1/4	$129.00	INCI

The California Nonprofit Corporation Handbook: computer edition with disk

ATTORNEY ANTHONY MANCUSO
CALIFORNIA 1ST ED.

This is the standard work on how to form a nonprofit corporation in California. Included on the disk are the forms for the Articles, Bylaws and Minutes you will need, as well as regular and special director and member minute forms. Also included are several chapters with line-by-line instructions explaining how to apply for and obtain federal tax-exempt status. This is a critical step in the incorporation of any nonprofit organizaton and applies to incorporating in any state.

IBM PC 5 1/4	$69.95	NPI
IBM PC 3 1/2	$69.95	NP3I
MACINTOSH	$69.95	NPM

How to Form Your Own New York Corporation: comuter edition with disk

How to Form Your Own Texas Corporation: comuter edition with disk

ATTORNEY ANTHONY MANCUSO

More and more businesses are incorporating to qualify for tax benefits, limited liability status, the benefit of employee status and financial flexibility. This software package contains all the instructions, tax information and forms you need to incorporate a small business, including the Certificate of Incorporation, Bylaws, Minutes and Stock Certificates. The 250-page manual includes instructions on how to incorporate a new or existing business; tax and securities law information; information on S corporations; Federal Tax Reform Act rates and rules; and the latest procedures to protect your directors under state law. All organizational forms are on disk.

NEW YORK 1ST ED.

IBM PC 5 1/4	$69.95	NYCI
IBM PC 3 1/2	$69.95	NYC3I
MACINTOSH	$69.95	NYCM

TEXAS 1ST ED

IBM PC 5 1/4	$69.95	TCI
IBM PC 3 1/2	$69.95	TC3I
MACINTOSH	$69.95	TCM

Two Years Free!

Nolo Press wants you to have top quality and up-to-date legal information. The **Nolo News**, our "Access to Law" quarterly newspaper, contains an update section which will keep you abreast of any changes in the law relevant to **Elder Care**. You'll find interesting articles on a number of legal topics, book reviews and our ever-popular lawyer joke column.

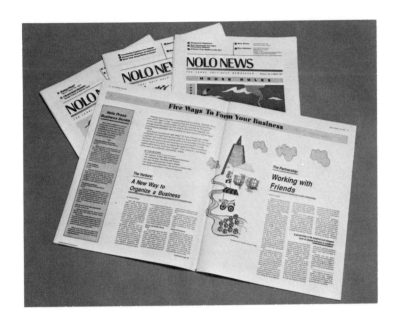

Send in the registration card below and receive FREE a two-year subscription to the **Nolo News** (normally $12.00). Your subscription will begin with the first quarterly issue published after we receive your card.

- -

NOLO PRESS
Elder Care Registration Card

We would like to hear from you. Please let us know if the book met your needs. Fill out and return this card for a FREE two-year subscription to the *Nolo News* (if you have already paid for a subscription, we will extend it for two years). In addition, we'll notify you when we publish a new edition of **Elder Care.** (This offer is good in the U.S.only.)

Name _____   Suggestions for improvement: _____

Address _____   _____

City _____ State _____ Zip _____   _____

Your occupation_____   _____

Briefly, for what purpose did you use this book?   _____

_____   _____

_____   _____

Did you find the information in the book helpful?   _____
  (extremely helpful) 1 2 3 4 5 (not at all)   _____

Where did you hear about the book? _____   _____

Did you consult a lawyer?_____   _____

Have you used other Nolo books?____Yes, ____No   _____

Where did you buy the book? _____   _____

▲

[Nolo books are]..."written in plain language, free of legal mumbo jumbo, and spiced with witty personal observations."

—ASSOCIATED PRESS

▲

"Well-produced and slickly written, the [Nolo] books are designed to take the mystery out of seemingly involved procedures, carefully avoiding legalese and leading the reader step-by-step through such everyday legal problems as filling out forms, making up contracts, and even how to behave in court."

—SAN FRANCISCO EXAMINER

▲

"...Nolo publications...guide people simply through the how, when, where and why of law."

—WASHINGTON POST

▲

"Increasingly, people who are not lawyers are performing tasks usually regarded as legal work... And consumers, using books like Nolo's, do routine legal work themselves."

—NEW YORK TIMES

▲

"...All of [Nolo's] books are easy-to-understand, are updated regularly, provide pull-out forms...and are often quite moving in their sense of compassion for the struggles of the lay reader."

—SAN FRANCISCO CHRONICLE

affix
postage
here

NOLO PRESS

950 Parker St.

Berkeley, CA 94710